P.C.

A Layman's Introduction to the Prostate Cancer Experience

By

David S. Wachsman

iUniverse, Inc.
Bloomington

P.C.
A Layman's Guide to the Prostate Cancer Experience

This book is the author's overview of the prostate cancer experience. Its intent is to provide information and insights to men who have been diagnosed with the disease. It does not purport to be a source of medical or psychological advice or recommendations for any individual or group of individuals and should not be taken as such. Medical, psychological or other advice or recommendations should come only from each individual's own doctor and/or mental health professional. Characteristics of individuals cited but not named in this book have been changed to protect their identity.

iUniverse books may be ordered through booksellers or by contacting:

iUniverse
1663 Liberty Drive
Bloomington, IN 47403
www.iuniverse.com
1-800-Authors (1-800-288-4677)

ISBN: 978-1-4620-1063-9 (sc)
ISBN: 978-1-4620-1062-2 (ebook)
ISBN: 978-1-4620-1064-6 (dj)

Printed in the United States of America

iUniverse rev. date: 6/15/2011

To Holly

ACKNOWLEDGEMENTS

This slim book could not have been written without the help of a host of people.

First among them is my wife Holly Hollingsworth, to whom it is dedicated. She has been a full partner at every medical meeting from the start. I could not imagine contending with this disease or writing this book without her unwavering support, uncanny insights, wisdom and love.

Also first among them is Yoshiya (Josh) Yamada, MD, FRCPC, a gifted radiation oncologist at Memorial Sloan-Kettering Cancer Center. (We all know that only one person can be first. This instance is the exception.) He studied my case, designed my treatment program and has managed the case ever since -- always with professional skills far beyond my understanding, with candor and with a robustly positive attitude. I will always be grateful for his care. This gratitude extends to members of Dr. Yamada's remarkable team: Joan Zatcky, RN, ANP and Elisa Mangarin. RN, BSN, OCN.

Thanks are due also to the many Sloan-Kettering physicists and other technicians -- from those who built the three-dimensional computer model of my prostate...to those who daily bolted me down to the treatment table with the aid of a hand crafted, plastic bas-relief of my nether end...to those who ran the computer program that directed the radiological beams to their target. And thanks to Regina Pineda, RN, BSN, who administered the monthly hormone shots that gave me new insights into what women experience in menopause.

For Dana Rathkopf, MD, singular thanks and eternal indebtedness for her professional care and personal compassion. My wife, Holly, my family and I have readily relied on the good doctor for her assiduousness, insight and gentle heart. No matter where--no matter when, Dr. Rathkopf has been there for us, carefully navigating our way through each twist and turn with expertise, understanding and strength .

I owe a special debt of appreciation to some good friends who started down the prostate cancer track before I did -- in a few cases long before -- or who joined me along the way. They are (alphabetically by last name) John, Lou, Bob, another Lou, Fred and Mac. Without exception, they've been open about their experiences. They've shared insights, answered questions and generally made the journey easier. Happily, all of them have conversed about this disease coolly and objectively, without undue fuss. Their support has meant much.

And this book could not have been written without an exceptional group of men who meet monthly under the aegis of Sloan-Kettering's Post-Treatment Resource Program. This workshop is open to men who have or have had any type of cancer. During the years that this book was being written, it was directed by an equally exceptional woman, Rachel Odo, MSW. She brought a rare gift of getting normally reticent men to express their deepest feelings to each other. With her colleague Richard Hara, Ph.D., MSW, she led exchanges of view on all the key aspects of living with cancer. Some of the most important insights in this book were first voiced by the uniformly courageous members of this group. I've tried to be true to their feelings and their words. Heartfelt thanks to them all.

Thanks to urologist John Coleman, MD for his invaluable insights. Thanks also to Stephen Connolly, MD and all those other doctors whose counsel and referrals meant so much and to those whose lectures Holly and I have attended. And to internist Wendy Ziecheck, MD, to friend and filmmaker Robert Geller and to others already named who took the time to review and comment on the manuscript. Any errors are mine, not theirs.

Milton Eisner, at the Cancer Statistics Branch of the National Cancer Institute, was generous as a key source of statistics, and he has my appreciation. So do James Carmody, Ph.D., Assistant Professor of Medicine and Director of the Research Center for Mindfulness at the University of Massachusetts Medical School; and Eileen O'Brien, an editor at the Health Publishing Business Group of Johns Hopkins Medicine. Both directed me to valuable information on diet. Appreciation also to friend Harris Hyman III, MD for his information on medical education.

All of these people understand that prostate cancer is terribly serious but can be talked about without a long face -- and even sometimes with humor. They recognize that it can allow, with luck, a great deal of living after treatment. I hope this book is, at least in a small way, worthy of them.

FOREWORD

by Mary S. McCabe, RN, MA
Director, Survivorship Program
Memorial Sloan-Kettering Cancer Center

Despite the fact that 230,000 men are diagnosed with prostate cancer each year, for the individual man and his family it is a unique, very personal journey. Beginning with diagnosis, there is immediately a tremendous amount of new information to be discussed, treatment decisions to be made and accommodations to be planned, both at work and home.

As health care providers, we try to provide our patients with accurate and complete information to assist in decisions and plans, but it doesn't include the same first-person viewpoint that comes from a man who has already been through the experience. This book provides exactly the kind of clear, insightful information that is needed. The author acknowledges the daunting task of handling fears and uncertainty and offers practical suggestions for dealing with them.

Included in the book are chapters that address how to navigate the medical system, as well as how to address the inevitable challenges of treatment. This step-by-step guide is a valuable resource to assist men through one of life's most difficult challenges in the prostate cancer journey. Congratulations to the author.

Contents

PREFACE

The initials P.C. are increasingly popular these days. They stand for personal computers, which are growing in number toward a possible one billion by 2010. They also stand for political correctness, which first became a subject of discussion only a decade or so ago and is now built into our language. Regrettably, they also stand for another growing phenomenon -- prostate cancer, a disease that one out of every six men will develop in his lifetime. This disease is, in fact, anything but politically correct. It's for men only. No exceptions. The reason is obvious: Men have prostates, and women don't.

If you've been diagnosed with prostate cancer, you're one of more than 200,000 Americans who each year unwillingly join a huge fraternity. By the start of 2007 (as of this writing, the most recent year recorded in detail by the National Cancer Institute), the membership stood at more than 2.2 million living American men who had been diagnosed with this disease and, in most instances, treated for it. (I'm reflected in that number because I joined the fraternity in 2000.) Our membership rolls appear to be growing. The 2007 figure was 1 percent higher than the year before.

As a group, we're as diverse as fraternity brothers can be, representing all ethnic, religious and economic groups and every state in the nation. A number of distinguished statesmen, business leaders, athletes, artists and other celebrities are fellow-members.

So are many hundreds of thousands of men whose names never show up in news media. Except for the fact that most of us are at or beyond the high end of middle age -- and the fact that representation of African-Americans is disproportionately high -- we are a solid cross section of male Americans. We have only one thing in common, and we'd much prefer that we didn't.

Being a member of this fraternity takes getting used to. If you're old enough to have prostate cancer, you may well be old enough to remember the bad old days when any kind of cancer was considered to be so grotesquely horrible that it was unmentionable. Even doctors talked around it by calling it "The Big C." The phrase "dread disease" was enough to tell you exactly which dread disease was being discussed.

Newspaper obituary writers usually omitted the usual cause-of-death reference when cancer was involved. Sometimes they discreetly cited "undisclosed causes" to assure that readers had no doubt. The still-current metaphorical use of the word, as in "a cancer on our industry," didn't help.

This long established view of cancer as always catastrophic and nearly always terminal has abated somewhat in recent years, as scientific research and medicine have combined to enlarge understanding of the disease. Diagnostic and treatment protocols have improved at an astonishing pace and continue to do so. As recently as the mid-1980's, cancer *survivorship* was not even a field of active study. Today, because so many people are living well beyond their cancer treatments, it has become a subject of intense interest at a number of institutions. Leading newspapers and newsmagazines have featured the subject on their front pages and covers. Cancer remains a feared, treacherous, potentially deadly disease, but great progress continues to be made. A lot of prostate cancer patients are doing just fine.

Whether or not you remember the bad old days of presumed hopelessness, a diagnosis of cancer in your own body can strike you as a devastating blow. It can bring to mind thoughts like *death sentence, nightmare, wasting away* or *egregious pain.* Thoughts along this line are not unusual when men first hear that they have prostate cancer, but there's no reason for you to conclude that they have anything to do with your case. They may very well not. For one thing, not all types of cancer are alike. Prostate cancer, for example, tends to develop more slowly than many of the others.

Still, applying the possessive to scary words – "my cancer" or "my tumor" -- takes getting used to. Be assured: As you learn more, as you advance through treatment and beyond, there's a good chance that the original fear built into these words will diminish for you. One day in the future, maybe sooner than you can imagine, you might find yourself using them in a totally straightforward, matter-of-fact way. Like many other men, you'll come to accept the reality that these words represent, not the *imagined* reality -- what they do mean, not what they could mean.

Obviously, however, prostate cancer is not just a medical matter. It is also a life matter. The first question all of us have to answer is, of course, "How am I going to get this disease treated?" Then comes the vital, ongoing question, "How am I going to live in this new situation?" Maybe you think of these questions as non-starters. *I'll get the damn thing dealt with,* you might decide, *and then live the way I always have.* It's possible that you will, but you're going to find that this disease is substantially different from others you may have experienced. A principal difference is this one:

Every cancer, including prostate cancer, metastasizes immediately upon diagnosis to the mind.

In other words, your mind is going to operate differently -- maybe only slightly but still differently -- from the way it did in the past. Some of your attitudes, beliefs and expectations are going to be challenged. If you were recently diagnosed, these changes have already started to take place. There's no cause for alarm here. You are and will continue to be definitively yourself. It's just that the old male sense of confidence and control that got you through so many earlier challenges might just come up short in the face of this one.

You know already that you are embarked on an exceptional journey in your life. Along the way, you're going to encounter some surprising non-medical situations that demand new ways of thinking. You're going to have thoughts and emotions you haven't experienced before. These changes can be subtle or profound -- or a combination of both -- but they're going to capture your attention. Your world won't be as topsy-turvy as Alice's after she dropped down the rabbit hole, but it will be different in important ways from the world you've known so well for so long. Many of the changes will be based on the way you and other people actually feel about cancer. Other changes will revolve around the reality that uncertainty has become one of the underlying aspects of your life. You can try to bull your way through it or deny it. You have a good chance of forgetting about it for long periods of time. Still, that uncertainty is not going away.

This book is the one I wish I'd come across when I joined the fraternity or soon thereafter. It takes a hard look at some of the non-medical issues you may not have thought about. If it has succeeded, you'll recognize them when they turn up in your life. You'll learn how some other men have dealt with them and get ideas about how you might manage them in your own way. Not least, you'll discover some new ways to think about your situation.

What this book is not about is treating prostate cancer. There are countless volumes on that topic. It's about dealing and living with prostate cancer; about handling unfamiliar situations that are going to arise; about regaining a sense of control; about living productively, well and, yes, happily to the outer limits of possibility.

DEALING WITH IT

IMAGINATION

The journey often starts quietly. You go for a checkup, and your internist or urologist finds one or two anomalies. Maybe a manual exam has shown that there's a rough edge or odd shape on your prostate. Maybe your PSA (prostate specific antigen, a blood factor that can signal the possibility of prostate cancer) has tested high or, whatever its level, has risen too fast. Maybe both. You're surprised. You've had no warning signal and feel just fine. You're in no way prepared to conclude that you have prostate cancer.

Neither is your doctor. He or she will suggest that you undergo a biopsy of tissue from several areas of your prostate to find out for sure. For many men, *undergo* means just what it says. They find it a terrible experience. Others find it much less distressing. They feel a series of sharp stings in the prostate while they're lying in a fetal position, certainly not a walk in the park but bearable. In either case, you may have a little blood in your urine for a few days after the procedure, but the doctor will give you advance warning about it and explain that it's no cause for alarm.

Here's the reality: The biopsy will prove unfavorable or probably favorable. Why *probably*? Because this important diagnostic procedure typically involves random samples of the prostate, and sampling errors are possible. In other words, a biopsy can miss the trouble spot. If you have a high or fast-rising PSA, it's still possible that cancer lurks in your prostate -- even

3

though your biopsy result doesn't prove the point. Your doctor will confirm the favorable reading or recommend the next step, which might include a second biopsy.

As you await an unfavorable or probably-favorable test result, you might find yourself thinking that the odds are about 50-50. Of course, they aren't; either you have a benign prostate or you have a malignant tumor right now. The odds are 100-100, but you don't yet know which 100 percent reality applies. The biopsy and the doctor's interpretation of the result are not going to change your prostate. They're only going to tell you what's going on, but knowing what's going on is extremely valuable. Once you do, you can either relax and get on with your life or deal with a very troublesome situation as well as you possibly can -- and still get on with your life.

The problem is not the biopsy process. The problem is waiting for the results of the biopsy process. You have the satisfaction of having done the right thing in the face of a potential problem, but your satisfaction is likely to be diluted by the Big Question: *What if the results should indicate prostate cancer?* Unless you're a man who never speculates about the next bridge until you come to it, your imagination is going to kick into overdrive at this point. The imagination at work here is not the kind that goes into telling stories, painting pictures, composing music or finding creative solutions to challenging problems. It's the unbidden kind that probes the future for possibilities. You might fantasize a clean bill of health. If so, enjoy it. You're more likely, however, to home in on the frightening *what if* question. Depending on your imagination's creativity, your life experience and your outlook -- and depending on how much your doctor has explained -- you

4

might picture yourself swiftly wasting away, putting on a brave face, your friends supporting you and telling you how good you look. You might see yourself in a hospital bed with a network of tubes keeping you going. You might even fantasize, for an instant, your own funeral, but you probably won't dwell on it. Your imagination can now have a field day.

This unruly, often misleading kind of imagination is most likely to come calling during occasional times like this one, when you're awaiting test results or you're between appointments. These are times when nothing seems to be happening and there's nothing much you can do. Like anyone who senses a crisis, you feel impelled to *do something right now*, but you've already done everything you can up to this point. It's only natural that your mind will tend to churn.

Imagination is a necessary component of your mental construct, and it can be wonderfully productive. In this case, however, your imagination lacks the vital resources it needs to be productive: data. Unless you're a doctor or medical student, or you've been very close to someone with prostate cancer, you simply don't know enough to imagine in a useful way. Your imagination may scare the hell out of you at this point, but it won't provide much guidance on what to expect.

If your doctor should conclude on the basis of all the evidence that you don't have prostate cancer after all, your relatively uninformed imagination will immediately become a non-issue -- if it ever arose in the first place. You'll recognize that you've dodged a bullet, count your blessings and possibly love your life even more than you did before. If it should turn out that you do have prostate cancer, on the other hand, you'll discover that your

5

doctor can rein in your imagination to some degree. He or she can explain the actual possibilities you face, often substantially different from the ones you dreamed up. Your doctor might not, however, talk to you about the things you fear the most, if only because there's no reason to believe that they will occur. It's never easy to reveal the things you fear most -- even to your doctor -- things that may appear to be totally unfounded or even silly. Ain't manly. Still, my advice is to ask. The doctor knows you're scared. Most of the men in his or her practice are frightened at one point or another. If your wife or partner is with you, she or he is scared, too, and will welcome the doctor's insights.

One idle thought that might pop into your head during this conversation is the matter of dying. If you have your own newly discovered cancer, it's hard to put the thought entirely out of your mind. While you are asking the doctor your initial questions, include one about this subject. It's not easy. Somehow you can't picture yourself asking the question hallowed by so many old, melodramatic movies: "Doc, how long have I got?" Fair enough. Change the language if you wish, but ask.

I did. It wasn't that hard for me. I happen to be someone who peers over precipices. Don't ask me why. I just like to find out what's down there. Then I do everything I can to avoid slipping over. Worst-case scenarios are also part of my profession, which frequently requires development of crisis-management plans. Looking at grim possibilities has become a habit.

I asked the urologist who discovered my problem about the possibility of a swift demise. I have since asked general oncologists, surgeons, radiation oncologists and other medical specialists about the issue. Based on their answers, as I understand them, here's a brief, simple overview of the situation:

Prostate cancer tends to develop more slowly than many of the others. In general, the older you are when it appears, the more slowly it tends to develop. It's best to catch it early -- a good argument for regular checkups. "Many men die *with* prostate cancer," doctors like to point out. "Far fewer die *of* it."

This final observation offers no guarantees, and it does raise the subject of mortality, but it gave me welcome relief when I first heard it.

In the months ahead, you're going to learn a lot about this disease and the medical methodologies for dealing with it. You'll realize one day that you're pretty knowledgeable on the subject, and you'll have a reasonable handle on your future, at least your foreseeable future. Even then, don't expect your imagination to shut down. It probably won't. It will more likely turn up from time to time as long as you live. From then on, though, it won't have the power it once did. There's nothing like knowledge to keep imagination under control.

PLUS AND MINUS

Speaking of your biopsy results, there's a medical-language anomaly that can cause you some momentary discomfort if you're not aware of it.

If you have previously had diagnostic tests that required interpretation or lab analysis -- X-rays, MRIs, CAT and other scans, biopsies, blood tests, urinalyses and others -- you already know that the language of the reports is counterintuitive. If you haven't, this usage may come as a surprise.

Subject to your doctor's interpretation, negative results are positive news, indicating that the test found nothing out of the ordinary. In other words, a negative report that's confirmed by your doctor is worth celebrating.

By the same token, positive results are negative news. To a greater or lesser degree, they indicate trouble. The only positive side to a positive lab result is the fact that a problem has been identified or confirmed and can now be dealt with. That fact is small consolation but considerably better than no consolation at all.

DECISIONS, DECISIONS, DECISIONS

When your biopsy results come back from the lab, the doctor will call you or, sometimes via his assistant, invite you in. A call is usually good news. A negative finding doesn't require a lot of explaining. Conversely, an invitation to stop by the office is usually less-good news. A positive finding in a prostate cancer biopsy requires a great deal of explaining. Still, don't let these speculations substitute for facts because there are exceptions. Some doctors like to share good news in person, and some prefer to get you over an initial shock by phone -- and then invite you in.

The actual results, as you know, will show that you probably have a clean bill of prostate health or that you have prostate cancer. If the results are negative and your doctor confirms them, count your blessings, get on with your life and continue your periodic checkups at the intervals the doctor prescribes. If the results are positive, make sure you get at least one additional piece of information, the rating of your tumor on what is known as the Gleason Score (or Grade). Dr. Donald F. Gleason years ago determined that the aggressiveness of prostate cancer cells could be graded on the basis of their configuration under a microscope. The neatest, most orderly cell patterns indicate the least aggressive, while the wildest, most disorderly ones point to the most aggressive. Dr. Gleason translated this finding into a scale from one to ten, from least to most aggressive. The way it works is this: A sample of malignant prostate tissue is given two individual grades on a scale of 0 to 5, one on the predominant pattern, the other on the background pattern. These ratings are added together, and the result becomes one's Gleason Score (or Sum).

A diagnosis of prostate cancer is obviously troublesome, but a low-to-medium Gleason Score moderates the misfortune. If you have such a score, then as a general rule all treatment protocols are open to you. I was a bit less lucky. I scored a nine. When I talk to anyone who's interested, I sometimes attribute my high score to the fact that I'm competitive by nature. In this case, however, there's a price to pay for a high score. I had originally opted for surgery, but no highly qualified surgeon would undertake my case because of that nasty nine. In retrospect, I have no regrets whatever that I was treated with conformal external-beam radiation and hormone therapy. Still, my radiation oncologist said it was heartening that the hormone therapy did what it was supposed to do (which is eliminate all one's testosterone and thus push one's PSA to zero). This therapy, it turns out, does not always work for Gleason nine cases.

Your mind might resist the report of a positive biopsy. *Couldn't the lab have mixed up my tissues with somebody else's?* If you simply can't accept the report, a second opinion is always an option. That said, odds are high that you will ultimately have to bite the bullet. The time will have come to accept reality.

Now you'll probably have that powerful urge to *do something, to deal with this thing.* Even if you're less decisive, you'll ask your diagnosing doctor a host of questions, and the doctor will answer nearly all of them. Along the way, he or she will spell out your principal treatment options. You'll learn that there are many different protocols and combinations of protocols for treating prostate cancer. While all of them can be effective, each one has its own characteristics and -- within these characteristics -- its own variables. These protocols include surgery, external-beam radiation, brachytherapy (radioactive seed implantation), hormone therapy, chemotherapy, cryotherapy, countless variations within each one and various combinations of modalities. Added to these treatment options is what the medical profession terms "watchful waiting." It's just what it sounds like -- consistent monitoring of the patient and no treatment at all. Some doctors conclude that when a man is especially old there's a good chance that another malady will catch up with him before his prostate cancer does. When you add to all these choices the huge number of medical institutions and individual doctors providing the various treatments, you realize the full scope of your choices.

The question the doctor will probably *not* answer is the very one you consider most urgent: "Which one's best for me?" There is simply no one-size-fits-all or even one-size-fits-most treatment plan. And because there is such wide diversity among the potentially effective treatment options, patient preference becomes an important part of the equation. Don't be surprised, therefore, if your doctor hands the decision to you. It's the usual approach. Suddenly you'll be introduced to a principle that applies to many aspects of the prostate cancer experience: "It's every man for himself." (There are few occasions when this phrase can be used without at least a few accusations of political incorrectness. This occasion is definitely one of them.)

"I'm not a doctor," I wanted to shout at this point. "I'm faced with the most important medical decisions of my life, and I'm in no way qualified to make them." In any event, I didn't shout. I just said it. The urologist had heard it before and understood, but he didn't back off.

"You don't know enough to make the decisions," he agreed. In other words, I'd have to learn everything I could about the various treatment protocols, make a choice, somehow evaluate doctors and their medical institutions and then make more choices.

"How much time do I have to find out everything I need to know and then start getting treated?" I asked.

"Well, you're not responding to a four-alarm fire here," he said. "The most important thing is to make the right decisions. You should take the time to do that." *Fine*, I thought, taking a deep breath. *At least I'm not under intense deadline pressure. I can approach this issue sensibly, deliberately.* But the urologist went on. "Of course, you don't want to take any longer than you have to." *Terrific.*

I was to hear this *you-don't-have-to-rush-but-don't-waste-time* construction often in the following weeks, as my wife and I talked to oncologists, surgeons, radiation oncologists, internists and other urologists. Predictably and I suppose responsibly, no one in the medical establishment would hazard a more specific reply. The doctors simply had no way of knowing. In the Brown v. Board of Education case, the U.S. Supreme Court mandated that the integration of schools be advanced "with all deliberate speed." This phrase, too, was imprecise but struck us as about right.

I was lucky. A friend of mine had undertaken the same research a year or two earlier and had saved every magazine article, health letter, web-site printout, booklet and book he'd studied before making his choice. He was good enough to lend me the collection, which arrived in a large corrugated box. I swiftly read it all, took thorough notes and thought of the process as Prostate Cancer 101. Then I went to many of the same sources and collected updated material. I was interested to note that medical science had not stood still. There were, in fact, new data and new protocols.

All this reading was prelude to the more important work – talking with the most qualified doctors we could meet in each of the treatment specialties. This intense research did what it was supposed to do: it brought my wife and me to the point at which we could make what felt like truly responsible decisions. How long did it take? Not quite six months. Was that too fast or too slow? Looking back, it seems about right to us. We couldn't have arrived where we did in less time and didn't need more. Would the same amount of research time be right for you? There's no way to know. It's every man for himself.

The more you learn, the more you will realize that, yes, treating prostate cancer *is* rocket science. There are few scientific and medical specialties that aren't involved. There are large numbers of variables that affect the outcome. A huge amount of technical and research data exists for each approach to treatment. Not least, knowledge of this subject is a moving target. Research is being advanced energetically; new knowledge is emerging; and some protocols are changing as a result. That said, the things you have to know to make an informed, prudent decision about your own treatment are *not* rocket science. You can learn them and understand them soon enough. A lot of men have.

As each of us has tried to do, you'll organize the research process that's best for you. There are some men who want to learn everything they possibly can, and there are others who prefer to know a lot less. Whatever your preference, however, you have to learn at least enough to choose a treatment protocol, practitioner and institution…to know why you made these choices…and to feel good about them. Here are a few brief suggestions. Some of them are expanded upon in the following chapters.

Overview

☐ Remember that time concerns in decision making aren't unique to men diagnosed with prostate cancer. Before attacking, generals and admirals want as much information about enemy resources and deployments as they can possibly gather. The more they can

13

find out, the more likely it is that an attack will succeed. On the other hand, if reconnaissance takes too long the optimum moment for a successful attack will pass. They have to find a balance between "learn all you can" and "move ahead" -- just as you do.

Prostate Cancer 101

☐ Read as much valid information on the basics of the disease as you can access. Validity is the key; so concentrate on sources that are unquestionably reliable. The ones I found especially helpful included the American Cancer Society, Atlanta, GA; Cancer Information Service™, a program of the National Cancer Institute (1-800-4-CANCER); Johns Hopkins White Papers, Palm Coast, FL; The Harvard Men's Health Watch, Boston, MA; and Mayo Clinic Health Information, Rochester, MN. Memorial Sloan-Kettering Cancer Center, New York, NY and M.D. Anderson Cancer Center, Houston, two leading cancer institutions, offer reliable information. There are, of course, numerous other good sources, and your doctor might well point you in the right direction to find them. Even if it were possible, there would be no sense in trying to tap them all. Your objective is not to become one of the world's leading authorities on prostate cancer. It's to gain an accurate, basic understanding of the disease so you can ask the most useful questions when you confer with doctors...and so you can make informed treatment decisions when you're ready.

☐ You can find valuable information on the internet if you're computer savvy, but restrict your search to unquestionably responsible sources. There's a large reservoir of total nonsense about this disease on the net. Some of it is smoothly, convincingly written, but it's nonsense nonetheless. Stay with the sites of highly regarded medical institutions or cancer- related service organizations.

☐ Be aware that your case may not be "average." (See the chapter titled *The Law of Averages.*)

☐ Ask your doctor and your leading local medical institution about any upcoming lectures or seminars on prostate cancer that you might attend. The medical professionals who speak at these events usually offer well organized information and insights. In addition, they often take questions as part of the formal program or afterwards.

☐ If you know other men who have been diagnosed and/or treated for prostate cancer, their insights might be useful to you. Never forget, however, that their cases can be dramatically different from yours. As a result, their insights might be misleading rather than useful. (See the chapter titled *Comparing Notes.*)

Beyond Prostate Cancer 101

☐ As you read and listen, jot down your questions as soon as they arise. (Have no doubt; they'll arise. You'll almost certainly want to know how certain general statements about the disease might apply to your case, for example -- or if they apply at all.) It's easy to forget questions, even important ones, when you're sitting with the doctor who can address them. Best to have them in writing.

☐ Cast as wide a net as you can to identify the leading specialists in each of the treatment protocols you're considering. Talk to the doctor who diagnosed your case, friends, someone at a local medical facility and other sources. The specialists have to be accessible to you, of course. If you live in a major city, reaching them should be no problem. If not, you may have to decide how far you're prepared to travel for the treatment you ultimately choose.

☐ Visit these specialists, tell them as much as you can about your case and find out as much as you can about each one's prostate cancer treatment protocol. You may be asked to bring any existing reports and/or scans to such meetings.

☐ If you possibly can, enlist a committed and, ideally, loving partner to join you in the process at this point -- wife, partner or genuinely caring friend. (See chapter titled *Building Your Team*.)

☐ Get optimum value from every medical appointment. (See chapter titled *Appointments*.)

☐ As you talk with doctors in each of the treatment specialties -- surgeons, radiation oncologists and others -- keep in mind that they tend to consider their own specialties the best. It's only natural. They wouldn't be in these specialties if they didn't believe in them. At the same time, most of these practitioners will steer you away if their protocols are obviously not right for you.

☐ When you have a clear sense of your treatment options, pick the protocol or combination of protocols that gives you the greatest confidence. Given a choice, go with a doctor who has done a lot of your selected procedures rather one who has done relatively few. And ideally, choose one who's associated with an institution that has an excellent reputation for its cancer-treatment service.

THE LAW OF AVERAGES

Look out for averages. As you read about prostate cancer -- in books, magazines, health letters or on the internet -- you're almost certain to encounter them often. They're fine as far as they go, but they can point to conclusions about yourself that may or may not be accurate. If your PSA, PSA-change and Gleason Count numbers are all on the low side, the averages that pertain to life expectancy and the chances of recurrence can be wonderfully reassuring. If one or more should be on the high side, on the other hand, these averages can be more than worrisome.

Case in point: When I was trying to get a handle on my own case soon after diagnosis, I came across numerous charts designed to predict the future of men with various Gleason Counts, from low to high. The counts rose on the left hand margins, and the average life expectancies went from left to right across the bottom of the page. It was impossible to miss that fact that most of the "lifelines" for low Gleasons moved crisply across the page, some almost to the right-hand margin. The lines for my Gleason 9, on the other hand, tended to stop about half way across the page -- or less. Accompanying words like "most lethal" or "most likely to spread" didn't help. At first glance, and for a while thereafter, these charts looked to me like a death sentence or, more accurately, a very-short-life sentence, until...

I realized that this chart, like most, was based not on any one case but on averages. Now, I have no quarrel with the value of averages. They provide useful insights. They help answer questions like, "What's the norm?" or "What's usual?" or "What's the situation in general?" What they don't do is serve as reliable predictors of individual cases. They can be encouraging or discouraging, but what they ultimately deal with are odds, not individual certainties.

As an example, let's say that you're a baseball fan. Your team has two on with two out. The next batter, representing the go-ahead run, has a solid .333 average. You know that this average makes him an elite hitter, one of the best on the team, and you have a sense of confidence as he takes his stance. Surprise! He strikes out. You remember that .333, a terrific batting average, means this player gets a hit only once for every three at bats. The odds were two to one against him this time.

Another example. Here are two columns of numbers:

11	20
10	14
10	10
10	5
9	1

The numbers in each column average ten. Obviously, the numbers on the left cluster very closely to the average. The ones on the right are all over the map. Both examples are somewhat extreme, but they make the point. Averages don't tell you much about an individual situation unless you know the spread of the numbers that were averaged, from highest to lowest. If the situation involves numerous variables, they mean even less.

Did I come to this viewpoint as a way of making myself feel better? I suspect so. I'd much prefer to have a Gleason below, say, 4 than the one I have. Still, I know two things that help sustain me. One is that prostate cancer is a complex disease with many variables, and every man's case is different from every other man's. The second is that the individual numbers that add up for an average can stray far from that average.

These two facts, taken together, don't give any of us a guarantee, but they give all of us a chance.

The law of averages was made to be broken.

COMPARING NOTES

You'll discover, if you haven't already, that we prostate cancer patients or veterans really are a fraternity. If you ask, most members will welcome the opportunity to share their experiences and insights with you. Many will be surprisingly forthcoming, specific and detailed in discussing their own cases. They might offer their understanding of general aspects of the disease, answer questions and make suggestions. They'll take the time to be as helpful as they can, treating you more like a brother than a stranger or just a friend. Their support can mean much.

While some of these men have a clear, accurate knowledge of the disease, however, others understand less, and still others offer information that is either out of date or outright wrong. Some of the personal experiences they share may prove wonderfully encouraging. Others may be seriously frightening. Be aware that their cases might have little or nothing to do with yours. As suggested in the previous chapter, the beginning of wisdom in your new situation is this:

From a medical standpoint, you are different from everybody else; your prostate cancer is different from everybody else's; your doctor is different from every other doctor; your treatment is likely to be at least slightly different from everybody else's treatment; and your outcome will be strictly your own.

Do prostate-cancer tumors have some similarities? Sure. A great deal is known about the way they behave, and certain treatment protocols are utilized often. Still, there are nearly always individual variations. Two of my best friends were treated with external beam radiation long before I was, for example. One warned of temporary incontinence, and the other reported serious rectal discomfort -- both during treatment. When my turn came, I waited for either or both symptoms to occur. They never did.

Another example: During my treatment, I spent a good deal of waiting-room time with men whose prostates were also being targeted by high-intensity radiation beams. I talked with many of them. There was wide variation in the number of their scheduled treatments. Some were simultaneously being treated with hormone therapy for various durations. Others were not. These men came from all walks of life and represented a wide range of ethnicities.

What they had in common were a small undertone of fear and a harmonious undertone of bravery, both so quiet as to be easily missed. We kept our conversations close to the surface, reached for humor and shared good cheer, much as I remember men doing in the army. Some of us compared notes about our treatments as a way of sharing and learning what we might. We enjoyed the connection but didn't learn much. It was obvious to all of us that we were new to this disease and that our medical situations were different -- just as they are among surgery and seed-implantation patients.

There are good reasons to compare notes with fellow members of the fraternity -- as long as you remember that the medical portion of these conversations may or may not be accurate or relevant to your case. It's undoubtedly interesting to share insights about life issues with fellow patients or veterans, and useful ideas often emerge. Here too, however, the circumstances, perceptions, feelings and styles of others might have little to do with yours. Perhaps the ultimate benefits of comparing notes are these:

☐ We discover that many of the problems, challenges and puzzles we face are not unique to us. We are not alone.

☐ We find that some of them really are unique to us. The way we deal with them will help define us.

☐ We gain insight into the infinite variety of ways that different men confront some of the same non-medical issues we face. In the process, we discover intellectual and emotional postures, practical steps and even tricks we can employ in our own lives.

☐ Not least important, we experience the unique pleasure of mutual support -- speaking candidly with someone who shares a vitally important personal situation and understands the underlying issues.

Unless you live in a sparsely populated area, it should not be difficult to find other men who are living with prostate cancer. The medical center or hospital where you're treated, or have been treated, can often direct you to a support group within reach. Equally to the point, you might be surprised at how many men you meet -- or already know -- have had experience with this disease. Some of them might welcome the chance to talk with you, and they represent a valuable resource of support.

But...

1. Remember again that other people's medical experiences are theirs, and yours will be yours. When it comes to the disease, itself, your doctor is far and away your most reliable authority.

2. You might be someone who strongly resists comparing notes with laymen. *Complete strangers?* you might think. *I shy away from discussing anything this personal with them. Is this something I really need to do?* No, it's not. You'll probably need support, possibly more than you expect, but other people in your life might give you all you need. If you have avoided sharing your feelings with strangers up to this point in your life, there's no compelling reason to start now. The cancer cells that have taken up residence in your prostate won't care one way or the other. If you've already

been treated, and any of those cells should remain in hiding, they won't care either. What matters are your own sense of what's right for you, your comfort and your commitment to pursue the medical protocol your doctor has laid out for you.

Fellow members of the fraternity can represent a genuine resource. It's available to you. Take advantage of it or skip it? The choice is yours. Once again, it's every man for himself.

BUILDING YOUR TEAM

We're men. We've been watching lone male heroes on the large screen and, more recently, small screen since we were kids. We've heard about them and read about them. We know that male heroes are tough, courageous and cool. When provoked or challenged, they battle back. Odds don't faze them. They take on big problems. They're self contained. They don't go running to mama. (Most of us are aware of female heroes, too, but, hey, we're men.) Think of private eyes like Philip Marlowe, Sam Spade and Spencer. Think of Frederick Douglass and Martin Luther King. Think of one-man armies like Achilles, Hector and Sergeant York. Think of the Lone Ranger, Gary Cooper on that empty street in *High Noon* and James Stewart in *Mr. Smith Goes to Washington.* Think of Superman, James Bond, Luke Skywalker and Frodo Baggins. Despite the evergreen popularity of "buddy movies," the spirit of the lone hero continues to loom large in our consciousness, and…

It's the last self image you should cultivate right now. Dealing with prostate cancer or any other cancer is a team enterprise. At its smallest and most obvious, the team is comprised of the patient and one or more doctors. Ideally, the team also includes a partner -- wife, lover, domestic partner, close relative, close friend -- someone who loves you, cares very much about you or is at least unquestionably on your side. At no time is this partnership more important than at the front end of the process, as you traverse the learning curve of treatment options.

(If there's no one in your life who fits the description, read on anyway. You might gain some insights into the issue, and your situation comes up later in this chapter.)

If you've just found out about your condition, you're about to undertake a comprehensive research program. To the extent that you can, you'll gather data by reading books, health letters and other materials; checking valid internet resources; attending any relevant seminars or lectures within reach; and talking with other members of the fraternity. Most important, you'll confer with doctors -- including those who specialize in the various treatment options. You'll assess your data and decide what protocol, doctor and institution will be best for you -- the ones that will give you the greatest sense of confidence. This task may sound more difficult than it is. Sure, it can involve a considerable investment of time and attention, but virtually any man can get his arms around the information he accumulates. Most of it is available in straightforward English, and no medical expertise is required for a basic understanding. Nevertheless, a committed partner can make the entire process easier and ultimately more successful.

Wait a minute, you might be thinking. *This won't be the first time I've gathered information and then made tough decisions.* You're right, of course. If you have ever chosen a place to live… or planned a vacation…or voluntarily changed jobs…or bought a new car or major appliance…or figured out an approach to your retirement plan, you've done this kind of work. This research project, however, is different in several ways. The need for this work probably came as a surprise and instantly rose to the top of your priority list. No matter how laid-back you might appear, you feel a sense of urgency, and it's appropriate. The discovery of this cancer has created a crisis in your life.

In a crisis, people behave differently from their norms, and most are completely unaware of the change. The only exceptions are police officers, fire fighters, military personnel, medical professionals and others trained and experienced in dealing frequently with crises. In a half-century-plus as a public relations professional, I have often helped companies and institutions respond to crises, including many that involved life and death. In the process, I've observed what happens: When a crisis strikes, the kind that costs or threatens human or even just business life, people separate from their own minds. Their reasoning function stops cold. Whether it's the chairperson of the board, the president or a down-the-line administrative assistant, shop steward or machine-tool operator, this effect takes place.

"We've got to *do* something!" is the most frequent reaction even before the shock of discovery wears off. It is most often accompanied by this one: "We've got to do it right away!" Only rarely do people react by saying, "Stop! We've got to think." As humans, most of us are just not built that way. Adrenaline kicks in. Our heart rate and other systems speed up; time seems to slow down; our awareness is heightened. All too often, people in a crisis do something, all right, but it's the wrong thing. It is specifically because panic severely curtails the ability to think rationally that cities, companies, schools and other organizations develop crisis-management plans and train their people in using them. Fire drills offer the most familiar example. Underlying virtually all these plans and training programs is the same simple message: "When you're suddenly faced with a crisis and 'have to *do* something,' do what it says in the crisis plan -- no more and no less."

What does all this have to do with me? you might be wondering. *I was shocked when I heard the diagnosis, sure, but I'm OK with it now. I can handle it without burdening anyone else.* Noble, but this crisis is not an event; it's an ongoing situation. You will probably encounter additional moments in which your crisis response takes hold. Not least among them are your meetings with doctors during the early months of your research and treatment, along with your checkups later. How could it be otherwise? Every one of these consultations will provide hugely important information about your personal future. Even if they don't involve imminent life-and-death issues, they may seem to. Result: You may not be at your absolute-best at these important sessions. Let me give you an example:

I had done a lot of homework before I had my first appointment with a major oncologist at a major institution. I knew my PSA and Gleason count, as well as the range of accepted treatment protocols. What I didn't know were "my chances." Sitting in the subdued, well populated waiting room with my wife, I realized that all these other people *had cancer*. Soon after, a routine reading by a medical technician showed that my blood pressure was elevated. Off the charts, to be specific. But I had no doubt that my mind was operating as well as ever. I was acutely aware of every detail of my surroundings and thinking clearly. No doubt about it.

We were directed to a small conference room with an impressively large, bright window. When the doctor entered in his well-starched, knee-length white jacket, he greeted us and sat in front of the window, which cast his face into partial silhouette. It was hard to read his facial expressions. He glanced at my charts, which had begun to accumulate and accompany me from appointment to appointment, and he proceeded to describe my situation. He didn't sound encouraging. He placed particular emphasis on my Gleason 9 and its precarious implications. I wondered aloud about the most effective protocols in these circumstances (having by now learned how to use the word *protocols* with reasonable proficiency). Instead of discussing the treatment options I had read about, however, he described an approach that included procedures I had never heard associated with prostate cancer. He explained them clearly, but they still sounded radical to me. "Your Gleason count," he explained. I thanked him, said I'd think about it, retreated from the meeting as swiftly as I courteously could, and decided never to deal with him again. He had scared the hell out of me.

It wasn't until evening, when my wife and I discussed the meeting, that I found out about the word I hadn't heard. "He said it was an experimental procedure," my wife said. "No, he didn't," I replied. She said she was certain and turned out to be correct. The doctor was recruiting participants for a test program, and I'd absolutely never heard the word *experimental*. She had. Any stranger monitoring that meeting might have seen me as entirely focused, thoughtful and even perceptive, but the reality was otherwise. Undetected panic had gotten in my way. That's the way it works. In these terribly important meetings, you sometimes hear what you want to hear, and you sometimes block out or rationalize what you don't want to hear. It's a perfectly natural reaction, but it can lead to mistaken impressions of important issues.

It isn't just me. I've heard from other people whose coolness I respect that they've had similar lapses in doctors' offices.

The lesson is obvious: Never attend one of these meetings with two ears if you can possibly listen with four. Who will bring the other two? As noted earlier, ideally your wife or partner or close relative or very best friend -- someone whose intelligence and judgment you respect. When such a teammate attends, you'll you be able to confirm later what you heard and understood, and you'll find out what may have slipped past you. Equally to the point, you will have somebody with whom to discuss whatever has come up, somebody who has the same body of information as you do. Discussions of this kind, even arguments when you're both committed to a successful treatment outcome, can help assure the most promising decisions. They are likely to increase your confidence in the choices you ultimately make. Not least, they might have the result of bringing the two of you closer together.

It goes almost (but not quite) without saying that the importance of a teammate's involvement never really diminishes. Your wife's or other partner's support is invaluable in infinite ways during your treatment, and it continues to be so in the months and years thereafter. There's rarely if ever a need to *lean on* your teammate, but there's enormous solace in simply knowing that this person "is there for you." (That obvious fact applies universally -- to men and women alike -- whether or not cancer has arisen in their lives.)

In short, it's perfectly OK to see yourself as a hero if it works for you. Just not a *lone* hero if you can avoid it.

But what if you can't avoid it? What if you feel there's no way you can deal with this process except alone? You could be in this situation for any of several reasons, including these:

☐ You're single, widowed or otherwise without an intimate or even very close relationship at the moment.

☐ You've been a loner for a long time, and you like it that way.

☐ Your wife or partner can't handle this challenge and doesn't want to think about what it might mean to you and your future together. The phrase "in sickness and in health" rings loud and clear in the wedding ceremony, but sometimes a marriage just doesn't work that way. The bonds can be stretched even more severely when there's no legal/spiritual commitment "as long as we both shall live." Dealing with the implications of cancer, for example, may seem like more than a relatively new wife or lover bargained for.

It is a troublesome reality that some relationships simply cannot bear the burden of a life threatening disease (and one that can result in brief or longer-term sexual dysfunction), even when the threat to life is modest or well into the future. Some loved people withdraw or actually leave. I have met men who suddenly found themselves alone at the very moment that they most needed warm, close support. The fact that these men represent a very small minority doesn't help you at all if you're one of them. If you are, your first imperatives are to survive the loss, to get through it and to regain or sustain the awareness of your own worth. Along the way, recognize this:

You could achieve a successful treatment without a partner if you had to, but you will never have to be alone in this enterprise. There will always be your doctor and members of his or her team, of course, and there will almost certainly be others you can engage if you want to.

If you want team support as you experience the trajectory of exploration, treatment and post-treatment life, now is the time to reach out. To whom? There are numerous possibilities. Here are some of them:

☐ **Family members and friends** -- OK, you may not want to share something this important and this *personal* with most of them -- or any of them, for that matter. And face it: If there are one or two you'd like on your team, they may not want to take on this responsibility. But recognize this fact, too: You may have a relative or friend who would be flattered by your invitation to become involved in your case. If so, you will have a loyal supporter. You'll still have the final say in every decision, but you'll have someone you know and trust with whom to discuss it.

☐ **Your internist, general practitioner or urologist** -- If your professional relationship is a long one, chances are it has taken on a personal dimension. (This doctor might even have been the one who first discovered your situation.) He or she might be a sophisticated, willing listener as you review what has taken place in your exploratory meetings with doctors and then sessions with your chosen treatment practitioner. Second guessing would not be helpful at this point, but this professional might at least serve as a good "sounding board." Naturally, fees would usually be involved. Only you can decide if such sessions are worth their cost.

☐ **Other members of the fraternity** -- Maybe you know people who have been treated for prostate cancer. Even if you don't know them well, many of them will be more than willing to listen, and they can be wonderfully supportive. You might derive great value in a personal connection with someone who knows the language of prostate cancer, and so might he, but remember the caveat in the previous chapter: No two cases are exactly alike. If you're concerned about something another member of the fraternity has told you, talk with your doctor or member of his or her team.

If you don't know any other members of the fraternity, they're not hard to find. Your selected doctor or other cancer specialists you've met during your search might be able to direct you to a prostate cancer group that meets periodically in your community. Social workers or other cancer-support professionals associated with local medical centers will usually have information on support groups.

The listings under *Cancer* in your local phone book might reveal organizations that can prove helpful, as can an internet search. (Reminder: Be especially careful on the web.)

☐ **Mental Health Practitioners** -- Psychiatrists, clinical psychologists, social workers, psychoanalysts and other therapists are trained in helping people under stress. They may not all be tuned to the realities of prostate cancer, but they do understand the issues of coping. Your chosen doctor's medical institution might offer the services of practitioners whose services are covered by Medicare and/or other insurance programs. Some other mental health professionals will also accept third-party payments. Most will not, and their fees can be high. In some communities, clinics offer the services of practitioners-in-training at low or moderate cost.

☐ **Members of the Clergy** -- Many people turn to their priests, ministers, rabbis, imams or other religious leaders (some of whom may be trained in pastoral counseling) in times of challenge. Like mental-health practitioners, these dedicated men or women might not be well versed in prostate cancer, but their insights into even larger life issues can be invaluable.

If *lone hero* is your style, if you have overcome every crisis in your life on your own, coolly and successfully, there's no inescapable imperative to change now. You could move ahead with a team of two -- your doctor and yourself -- and still get the job done. But if it occurs to you that now might be a good time to involve other people in your situation, you can find them. After all, that's what a fraternity is for.

If, on the other hand, you already have a loving partner in this enterprise -- along with good, supportive friends -- think about reaching even further out. You might find some of these additional resources to be invaluable. You might discover that they give you an expanded sense of vitality, well being and optimism. They've done it for me.

APPOINTMENTS

Some men see the relationship between patient and doctor as pretty much the same as the one between driver and auto mechanic. In either case, they think, the professional knows how the machine works, how to diagnose problems and, most important, how to fix them. If this professional has a good reputation, you can trust him or her to come up with the right solutions and do nothing that isn't necessary. You take the machine to the professional, and the professional takes it from there. Your only job is to pay, and it's worth it.

Not really, and certainly not now. The analogy is way off the mark.

In the case of prostate cancer, the relationship between patient and doctor is anything but one sided. It may not be an exactly equal partnership, but both parties have responsibilities. If either side fails to meet them, the chances of a true "fix" are greatly diminished. Let's look first at the doctor's responsibilities.

He or she has to maintain a current, encyclopedic knowledge of the human body and a deep understanding of how it works...has to understand the complex facts and nuances of prostate cancer in general and your case in particular...and needs an intimate understanding of the many available therapies and combinations of therapies. He or she must know how to develop the optimum treatment plan for you...how to modulate its various aspects with insight and precision...how to evaluate your progress...and how to work with you effectively as an individual. Most important, the doctor has to assume responsibility for treating you and keeping you informed. That's one side of the equation, and it's a tall order.

The other side is yours, and it's also demanding. It starts with knowing as much as you realistically can about prostate cancer, your own case and the various treatment options. By "realistically," I mean taking into account that you will always be a layman on this subject (unless you happen to be a physician or you're engaged in medical research or education). You have to know at least enough to understand what your doctor says, to ask questions that will contribute to your further understanding and to make a few major decisions. That's a lot, but it is not all.

Another of your responsibilities, even more important than the first, is to follow your doctor's instructions assiduously. That task will be easier if you understand them in the context of your individual situation and the disease in general.

You will owe it to yourself at some point -- you can ask your doctor when -- to explore and possibly take advantage of complementary therapies. Note that "complementary" implies *in addition to* your treatment, as opposed to "alternative," which indicates *instead of.* Exercise programs, massage, yoga, meditation, diet or vitamin options, psychological counseling and/ or other techniques might contribute to your treatment and are likely to contribute to your feeling of well being. It's a good idea to check with your doctor or another member of your treatment team before undertaking any such therapies.

Finally, you have a full measure of responsibility for making every appointment with your doctor as productive as it can possibly be. This responsibility starts now and will continue for as long as you can imagine. Don't think for a moment that you can just sit passively in the consulting room and let the doctor "take care of you." Here a few ways to do your share.

☐ **Write down your questions as they occur,** even if it's weeks or months before your next appointment. When they arise in your head, get them on paper, no matter how silly you think they might be to the doctor. Why? Because some of them are likely to vanish if you don't…and then rush back after the appointment. (How many times have you left a doctor's office thinking, *Damn! I forgot to ask about…?*) It can't hurt to date your questions as you go. Don't worry about how long your list grows. You'll discover that some of the questions are redundant and others can be grouped. Equally to the point, the doctor may well be aware of your most important questions before you ask them and knows how to provide the answers clearly and more briefly than you might expect. Still, be sure he or she answers all the questions you bring.

☐ **Arrive for your appointment on time.** The doctor almost certainly operates on a tight schedule, and disrupting it won't endear you to him or her. That said, be prepared to wait. This suggestion might seem contradictory, but medicine is not always a predictable profession. Every case, including yours, is different, and some require more time than could possibly be foreseen.

A doctor often makes pain-or-comfort and sometimes life-or-death decisions. Some require more data and take longer to make than others. If your doctor takes whatever time is necessary for some other patient, keeping you waiting at some point, count your blessings. You can expect the same deliberate care for yourself. It's a good idea to arrive with a book, magazine, newspaper or whatever, just in case. The magazines in most medical waiting rooms were last up-to-the-minute three or four weeks ago.

☐ **Take the question** *How're you doing?* **seriously.** Asked by family and friends, this question can be a modest courtesy. A simple *Fine, thanks.* is entirely adequate. When your doctor asks it, on the other hand, it is a diagnostic probe. He or she really wants to know how you're doing and, also important, how you describe what's happening. Your answer gives him information in two areas of interest: how you are and who you are.

☐ **Be yourself.** For example, don't use the appointment to show the doctor how tough or stoic you are -- unless you really are tough and stoic. Better to be exactly who you are: anxious, hopeful, determined, downright scared, calm, confident -- or, if they apply, any or all the above. As it is for so many interactions, honesty is the best policy. If you want to impress the doctor, do it by answering his or her questions accurately and completely, listening thoughtfully, asking your questions clearly and following instructions. If the doctor gives you a sense of confidence, it doesn't hurt to share that fact with him or her.

☐ **Be absolutely candid.** The doctor's office is the last place to keep secrets or avoid topics that make you uncomfortable. Keep in mind, for example, that the doctor and any nurses or other practitioners in the room know all about sex, urination and defecation. No matter how shy you may be about raising these topics in all other conversations, feel free to raise them here. Any one or all three can relate directly to your prostate cancer and treatment.

Just a second, you might be thinking. *Maybe that stuff is OK for the doctors or nurses, but you urged me to bring my wife, partner or friend to every medical meeting. Does this person really need to hear this stuff?* To be honest, that question gave me pause. It isn't exactly romantic to talk in front of your wife about erections, urine and stools. But if something odd is happening to you, something that might be important, maybe your teammate shouldn't be kept in the dark. That's what I decided, and my wife understood. If you much prefer the alternative, asking your teammate to step outside the room when these things are discussed, by all means do it. Note that this choice isn't perfect either.

☐ **Find out what you need to know.** Be sensitive to the time pressure on your doctor, but balance it with your need to know and understand what's happening. You're the patient, and awareness is part of your treatment. Keep your questions sensible and specific, but don't worry about what you think might be "dumb" ones. Sometimes those lead to particularly valuable answers. You can even ask questions that demand prognostication, but be aware that you are unlikely to get simple, straightforward answers. "Do you think I can count on 15 or 20 good years after this treatment is over?" you could ask, but don't expect a crisp "yes" or "no" response. Your doctor doesn't know -- and can't at this point. He or she might give you a well informed impression of your situation, but anything further would be a guess.

☐ **Take notes.** A lot transpires in even a short meeting, and it's very hard to remember it all. To put it the other way, it's easy to forget something important the doctor said -- or not to hear it at all. You don't want to guess what it might have been. I'm aware that "take notes" is not an easy suggestion to follow. Listening demands concentration. So does good note taking. If you have done it before, you've learned how to divide your attention between the two. If you haven't, just do your best and limit your notes to the most important points. Better yet, if someone has come to the appointment with you, perhaps she or he can take the notes.

Some people use bound notebooks for this note taking; others prefer loose-leaf binders; still others, any kind of pad. I opted for a ruled yellow pad and usually type up my notes when I get home, dating them and filing them in a folder in reverse chronological order. Accurate content matters much more than format, but choose a system that will enable you to save these notes. The process you've begun will not end after an appointment or two but will continue, if you include checkups, for the rest of your life. Even though the doctor will have a complete, detailed record of your progress, it's sometimes helpful to look back at your own data, not just for practical purposes but also to see where you've been. How about taping the meetings? I'd check with your doctor first. Physicians pay exceedingly high premiums for malpractice insurance, and one of them might understandably answer your questions with greater reserve than usual if you're recording. With extremely rare exceptions, doctors are committed to telling the truth to their patients, but your taping could be misunderstood. If you think listening to a replay of the meeting will be helpful to you later -- and your physician does, too -- there's no reason not to go ahead.

☐ **Debrief after the appointment**. You've just heard a lot, all of it important. Chances are you've been at least a little tense. Now the tension eases, and, almost inevitably, questions arise: *What did he say?*...or *Didn't she say something about (whatever)?*...or *Did he explain what would happen if...?*...and countless others. When you get home or to a nearby coffee shop, expand on your notes and try to remember what you were told. If a teammate was there with you, confer. Reach as many conclusions as you can. Only at that point will you have derived optimum value from the appointment.

The door hasn't closed when your meeting is over, of course. If you have an open question, one that you never asked or the doctor never answered -- and if it's important to you -- you can always direct it back to the doctor by phone either directly or via a nurse, nurse practitioner or other member of your treatment team. The same opportunity applies if you're troubled by an unexpected symptom, even if it occurs weeks or months after your most recent appointment. Worry contributes nothing to your treatment or your life, and there's no need to endure it any longer than necessary.

Yes, your doctor is your expert consultant and healer. Yes, he or she knows much more about prostate cancer and your particular case than you ever will. Yes, he or she has had experience in treating this condition. And yes, he or she has institutional resources -- colleagues and staff, research and testing support, facilities and equipment, and a body of systems and procedures, along with institutional memory -- that will help give you an optimum outcome. But you're not off the hook. As noted, you can't just turn the whole matter over to your physician and forget about it. You have a major role to play in this venture -- learning, understanding and questioning when you're in doubt -- in short, actively participating. My wife, who has had her own bouts with cancer, puts it this way: "When your health is involved, you have to be your own advocate." She's right. Knowing what the doctor is doing...why and how the doctor is doing it...what effect the treatment is having on you...and what kind of progress you're making will go a long way toward supporting your sense of control. This involvement will put you in a position to report your symptoms and reactions clearly and accurately. It will enable you to pose perceptive questions and to understand the answers. It will give you an idea of what to expect.

You don't have to invest an enormous amount of time to be an effective member of your own team, but you do have to invest some. Unlike many other investments, this one is almost certain to produce a valuable return.

OTHERS

A patch of green-carpeted floor reminded me of an important reality. I first noticed it in the airy, fourth-floor waiting room of Sloan-Kettering's radiation-oncology wing, where I received my daily doses of external-beam radiation. This patch cannot be identified by a pattern in the carpet or a stain or even a precise location. In fact, the location is different for each waiting-room chair. In general, it lies about four or five feet in front of any given chair, but it can be elsewhere.

This patch of floor does not exist until someone gazes at it for a long time, and it fades into the rest of the floor as soon as that person looks away. Let me explain.

When a prostate cancer patient who chooses radiation settles into the routine of daily treatments, he's likely to see a number of other patients often. Some of them have different types of cancer, but they are on roughly the same radiation schedule he is. As described in the chapter titled *Comparing Notes*, the patient tends to form light, sometimes candid and nearly always brief relationships with some of these people. With others, he simply shares a good wish or encouraging word.

One of these others was a tall, athletic-looking man who inevitably arrived in a well-cut gray or blue suit and discreet tie. He radiated a warm, bluff accessibility, behind which I detected a secure sense of command. A CEO, perhaps, or a partner in a Wall Street law firm. He was almost always accompanied by his wife, who appeared to be an almost perfect match. She, too, was tall. Her long legs, high cheekbones, masterful makeup and coif

-- along with her clothes, always a notch above fashionable -- suggested that she was or had been a model. In the waiting room, these two were intensely close, and she smiled often. Their hands were joined, and their heads were nearly always tipped together as they shared quiet conversations. Other patients couldn't help noticing them but maintained the distance that the couple evidently preferred. I sometimes met the husband in the changing room just before or after his treatment, and we exchanged pleasant, always positive greetings.

One day, at an hour when the waiting room was nearly empty, a radiation oncologist came out of the office corridor and joined the couple. The doctor, in the usual white coat, pulled his chair around to address them and held his hands together palm to palm. All three leaned in so they could talk quietly. I was far away and moved farther to expand their area of privacy. I did not hear a word, but a quick look at their expressions left no doubt that the conversation was a sober one. I busied myself with the book I'd brought, separating myself even further from the scene. Finally the doctor and the tall man rose, walked across the waiting room and vanished behind the door to the treatment area. I glanced over to where they had been.

That was when I first noticed the patch of floor. The comely wife was staring at it. Her smile, even the possibility of smiling, had vanished. Her eyes were misty, and a deep furrow had formed between them. Her head sagged forward; her mouth was slightly open, and a few strands of hair had fallen over one eye, as if all her supportive energy had drained away. I guessed that she did not see the patch of floor. Her gaze rested there, but it was clear that she was seeing far beyond it. It was easy to believe that she

42

was trying to envision the future and that a forest of frightening *what-ifs* was obstructing her view. She almost radiated the feeling of being terribly alone. Her eyes did not stray from the spot.

I met her husband later, after his treatment. He was back in his suit, leaving the changing room as I was arriving.

"How are you doing?" I asked.

"This has not been my best day," he said in a lower-than-usual voice.

I said at the start of this chapter that a patch of green-carpeted floor reminded me of an important reality. This is the reality: We prostate cancer patients are not the only ones wrestling with occasional fear, distress and possibly even moments of despair. For many of us, there is someone else who is suffering too, though she or he seldom lets us notice. Our wives or partners or closest friends sometimes stare at their own patches of floor when we are well out of sight. When these people are with us, they are nearly always cheerful, optimistic and even confident -- or so they make us believe. In their unflagging support, they are every bit as heroic as we may think we are.

If you have recently been diagnosed, just tuck this reality away for future reference. You are the patient, and you really do need support at this point. If you're lucky enough to have it, accept it graciously and with pleasure. At some point, however -- and sooner is better than later -- it will be important to remember that you are not the only one affected by this encounter with prostate cancer. You are not the only one wrestling with all the troubling, sometimes scary, new questions about your future. Your wife or friend is on the same journey and needs hopeful, loving support just as much as you do. You will not add to your burden by giving this support. You will lighten it.

LIVING WITH IT

ATTITUDE

"I'm going to beat this thing."

Most of us have encountered at least one cancer patient who's made this brave, gritty declaration -- in a movie, magazine or book, in a television interview or in real life. We live in a determinedly optimistic society, one in which a fighting spirit is given especially high priority. It's no wonder that large numbers of men with prostate cancer take it for granted that this unwaveringly positive attitude is a requirement for successful treatment. They assume that any other response risks a poor outcome; so they take on the heavy responsibility of "staying on the bright side." Convinced that it's best for their families and friends as well as themselves, they undertake a life-and-death struggle against fear, sadness, discouragement and gloom. For some men, this response is exactly right. They've honed it to a sharp edge while dealing with other challenges over the years. It fits them.

But it doesn't fit everybody. All of us have faced serious difficulties, and each of us has developed his own way to cope with them. One man's way might look like an ardent, uninterrupted, absolute belief in success, sure. Another's might involve stoicism, anger, a quiet commitment to do battle, simple determination, prayer, wishful thinking, a bedrock of hope, pursuit of a spirit of normalcy, a measure of denial or other approaches. Still another's way might involve a combination of responses and undergo a series of changes as the effort advances. And yes, some men have even experienced times of fear, sadness, discouragement and gloom while confronting difficulties and still done everything necessary to overcome these difficulties.

The tiny cancer cells that take up residence in a man's prostate don't appear to give a damn what the man's attitude is. There's no current evidence that says otherwise. What they do react to is the treatment that might remove them, kill them or beat them into a deep sleep. (In this respect, they're a little like the cartoon insects in bug-spray commercials. They cringe, scatter or die only when the spray is applied.) Do these facts indicate that your attitude doesn't matter? Not at all. It matters in three vitally important ways:

1. Your attitude must support -- or at least not get in the way of -- your doing your post-diagnosis homework and making your treatment decisions in an effective, timely way.

2. It must support -- or at least not get in the way of -- your following your treatment protocol to the letter and pursuing any complementary therapies you and your doctor agree might be helpful.

3. It will have a profound effect on the quality of your life and the lives of those around you. There's no need for an enthusiastically-upbeat-no-matter-what approach to life. Most people have occasional down periods while they're dealing with major challenges and even afterwards. There are moments when rage, disappointment, bitterness or a sense of mourning can be normal

parts of the process. Fine, as long as they're temporary. If they persist -- if they mutate into depression -- they can make your life and your world appear bleak and hopeless. The cancer cells may not be affected, but you and those who care about you are. As you may know, depression generally responds well to professional treatment.

To my knowledge, no one in the cancer-treatment universe has brought the role of attitude into clearer focus than Jimmie Holland, MD in her magisterial *The Human Side of Cancer* (written with journalist Sheldon Lewis and published in 2000 by HarperCollins.) Dr. Holland holds the Wayne E. Chapman Chair in Psychiatric Oncology at Sloan-Kettering and is professor of psychiatry at Weill Medical College of Cornell University.

When I first came upon this invaluable book, I was certain that the spirit inherent in "I'm going to beat this thing" was absolutely necessary to my survival. Still, I had a problem: I'd heard of people with this spirit who had lost to cancer and others without it who had won. More to the point, I couldn't summon the consistently rah-rah feeling for myself. It didn't fit. I was trying to root my approach in realism, commitment to doing the right thing, cheerful normality whenever possible and a modest aspiration to something at least a little like bravery. This attitude did fit, but it still worried me.

Imagine my reaction when I saw the title of Dr. Holland's second chapter, *"The Tyranny of Positive Thinking."* It's rare that a chapter title, alone, can have a profound effect, but this one did. Seeing it gave me an immediate pulse of liberation, even celebration. I had been doing it my way, and now an unimpeachable source made it clear that my way -- and anybody else's way -- was perfectly OK as long we were doing the work of pursuing the most successful possible treatment.

LUCK

Serious gamblers know a lot about luck. If you are among them, you know perfectly well that the odds are in favor of the house. (Taking the long view, the odds are in favor of the house in life, too. Who ever kept his or her winnings forever?) Still, whether for pleasure or addiction's sake or both, gamblers seek to defy the odds. They often analyze and plan in enterprises that don't necessarily lend themselves to analysis and planning. They push their chips or money out onto the table or their cash across the lottery-ticket counter or through the window at the track, ever hopeful that they will get lucky. They perceive "runs" of good luck and bad luck. Once they bet, their treasure is out of their hands. They've surrendered it to chance. They can root, but they can no longer do anything to affect the outcome.

Getting prostate cancer is bad luck, no question about it. To be strictly accurate, it may not be entirely a matter of luck. Family history is almost certainly a factor, and there may be lifestyle influences that have not been identified yet. Whatever the cause, however, things would have been better if this disease had passed you by. In other words, bad luck.

Always remember, though, that this particular instance of bad luck doesn't mean that your good luck has run out. It hasn't.

The very fact that you *know* you have prostate cancer is a clear instance of good luck, especially if your discovery has come early. It means you can do something about this situation. You can get it treated or, if you have your reasons, decide not to. If you choose treatment, you surrender relatively little to chance. Medical science plays a much larger role. There are no sure things, but your outcome is at least partially in your hands.

You are also the immediate beneficiary of another stroke of good luck. In most cases, cancer of the prostate is distinctly preferable to cancer that might have turned up in almost any other part of your body. As noted earlier, it tends to develop more slowly, and the older you are the slower the development. And you are joining this fraternity now instead of a long time ago. Medicine is advancing. New treatment modalities are being tested, and many have proved to be effective. This progress has been relatively rapid. Nerve sparing surgical techniques have been refined in recent years. So have radiation-delivery techniques. Even during the nine consecutive weeks of my treatment, a detail of the protocol was changed for the better. In other words, you have the benefit of all the progress that has been made and that continues. Do not misunderstand. I am not suggesting that your having this disease is anything but damn unfortunate and distressing. What I am saying is that it isn't the last luck you will have.

No one can predict with certainty how successful your treatment will be, but the odds are strong that you will encounter some good luck as you progress. Try to recognize it when it turns up, not always an easy task under the best of circumstances. If you have been a pessimist for as long as you can remember, it's an even more difficult task. Nevertheless, spotting, acknowledging and celebrating any good luck that occurs will be good for your morale and that of those around you. Doing so will also enhance your motivation to do everything your treatment protocol requires and, if you choose, even more in the form of complementary therapies.

In the final analysis, it is your treatment that deals with your tumor. Your morale deals with your life. When you notice good luck, you discover hope, and that's the key ingredient of high morale.

WHOM DO YOU TELL?

I can imagine your wondering why this question is even raised. The answer couldn't be simpler or more obvious: *I'll tell anybody I feel comfortable about telling.* This response is ultimately the right one. Keep in mind that your appearance and demeanor are probably going to be much the same as they were before your diagnosis; so it's unlikely that you'll be under pressure to explain visible changes. Your thoughts about reporting the news might be along these lines:

Your wife or partner or best friend almost certainly knows already. Depending on circumstances, you will probably want close relatives to be aware, but there may be a few you do not want to burden with the news. Friends? Chances are that you will want the close ones to know. You have every reason to expect them to be supportive. After all, support at times like this is part of what friendship is about, right? You may not feel impelled to advise more distant friends or acquaintances unless the subject comes up. Tell business colleagues or fellow workers? Well, that decision might require a little more consideration.

These thoughts may or may not reflect your own, but let me assure you that there is nothing simple or obvious about deciding whom to tell. The news of your prostate cancer is fundamentally different from anything you have ever told relatives, lovers, friends or fellow workers in the past. It is likely to elicit at least a few unexpected reactions.

☐ One man in treatment for prostate cancer told me this: "I met a good friend on a street corner, and we got to talking. When I told him about my diagnosis, he actually took a step back. It was impossible to miss. He was sympathetic, but he immediately put more space between us. He hasn't raised the subject since."

☐ Another telephoned his brother, who lived out of state, to tell him that he was going into treatment for prostate cancer. His brother expressed surprise and concern and wished him a good outcome. Based on their reasonably close relationship over the years, the patient expected at least a few calls from his brother to check on his progress and maybe to offer some cheerful wishes. The calls never came.

☐ A third returned full time to his construction job after treatment and discovered a change in his co-workers. He felt fine, he told them. "They were very friendly, but they treated me as if I couldn't handle any of the strenuous parts of my job. I explained to them that I could, but they kept on being *careful* with me. Another curious thing is that none of them would touch me -- no hand up from one level to another, none of the usual high fives or pats on the back. They must have thought it was catching."

My own experience has been twofold. I am blessed with a loving family and good, long-time friends, including five who have experienced prostate cancer. My wife has been my loving, committed equal partner in dealing with this disease from the moment my urologist first expressed concern. A few of my relatives and friends have wanted to know as much as I can tell them about prostate cancer in general and my case in particular. They, too, have been involved, sensitive and supportive. "How are you doing?" can be an easy throwaway question, but these people occasionally ask it in a tone that means they want a real answer. At the same time, they never press if I opt not to reply in detail. As I said, I am blessed.

On the other hand, there are others I've told who never purposely open the door to the subject. They would rather tell me how good I look than ask me how I feel. They would toss out at least a quick "sorry to hear it" or "you sound awful" as if I had a bad cold, but not a word on this subject. There is absolutely no fault here. These are good people. It is simply important to them to stay as far as possible from this aspect of my life. It's as if my prostate cancer were a sealed room, and, in early 21st Century parlance, they "won't go there." They haven't changed. Our relationships seem the same, too, at least on the surface, but they have undergone subtle adjustments. For the first time, some of us have discovered limits to how close we can be.

What's going on here? There's no single answer, but here are a few factors that appear to be at play. They do not, of course, apply to everyone.

☐ Some relatives and friends will react to your news exactly as you would hope -- with concern and genuine interest. You'll know immediately that they will be neither pushy nor distant, that you can count on their "being there" for you. Be aware, however, that they might be uncertain about the best way to be helpful. Should they assure you that you'll be fine? Should they check often on how you're feeling so you know they care? Should they treat you as if you'd like everything to continue normally, or should they look for new ways to make things easier or more pleasant for you? The fact is that they may not know for sure. You may have to guide them.

☐ You will usually find a sympathetic ear also when you talk with other men who have faced prostate cancer. If they are behind you on the track, you might help them with your new insights. If they are ahead, you might learn something useful from them. You know by now that all cases are different; so listen openly and sympathetically but also critically to your new fraternity brothers.

☐ There will be other people whose reactions strike you as puzzling. Most of those with whom you will share the news know a lot less about prostate cancer than you already do. They will be as frightened for you as you might have been when you first heard the diagnosis. After all, most of them have done absolutely no homework on the subject. They may have grown up in the days when "the Big C" was too deadly and acted too swiftly even to be named. You know better by now, but these people may suddenly see you as doomed, a family member or friend soon to depart forever. They are thunderstruck and terribly sad. They will probably try to cover up these feelings and might even assure you that you'll do fine, but they think they know better.

☐ Your news might make some people feel more vulnerable to cancer than they ever thought possible.

When it comes to all the hazards we could possibly encounter, most of us feel secure about the ones that haven't even come close. Because we haven't faced these hazards personally -- and nobody we know well has ever had to deal with them -- we feel insulated, protected. We sense from experience that the odds of these hazards ever confronting us are infinitesimally small. Now you come along with your news, and suddenly the odds seem to rush higher for those you tell. *If cancer can strike him, somebody I know, it could happen to me,* they might sense. When most people first hear about your situation, they hear the word CANCER in large capital letters and the word prostate in very small lower-case letters, if at all. In other words, your news might frighten some people, though they will generally do their best to cover it up.

☐ There are others who just can't handle being close to any kind of sickness. A heightened awareness of their own vulnerability might be part of it, but there's more. They feel viscerally threatened by even a non-communicable condition such as yours. For them, being physically close to someone with a medical problem, not to mention touching him or her, stirs the fear of "catching it." They may be aware that this fear is irrational, or they may try to rationalize it. In either case, they experience it.

☐ Some of the people you tell may see you in a different light. To them, you are now first of all a man with a life threatening disease. They see you as needing deference and freedom from undue stress and strain, along with new levels of sympathy. They might presume that, even after treatment, you will be weaker or your life expectancy will be much shorter than in the past. These views are uninformed, and none is likely to be valid, but the people who hold them will need convincing.

Unless you are retired, it could be your employer, colleagues or co-workers who see you in this changed light. If so, the issue of telling them is complex.

Do you want them to know?

Would you be comfortable if they did not know, if they believed that nothing had changed?

Do you even have a choice? Will the treatment protocol you select require that you explain your need for time off?

Are you concerned that, out of kindness, your supervisors, colleagues, customers or clients might be inclined to reduce your responsibilities or hold you to a lower standard?

The answers to these questions depend entirely on your own feelings and your sense of the people with whom and for whom you work. Take your time. If you have recently been diagnosed, you probably aren't ready even to consider these questions -- nor do they need answers right away. The good news is that you have weeks and possibly months to decide how to deal with them.

And keep this in mind: The issue of telling or not telling people about your prostate cancer is relevant but strictly secondary. The primary goal is to deal with your medical condition in the most effective possible way. The protocol you choose should be the one that you believe in your heart will be the most successful, the one that gives you the greatest confidence in the outcome. No other factor should color your decision.

☐ Here's a fact that's easy to overlook: When you tell people you have prostate cancer, you are presenting them with a new responsibility -- whether you mean to or not. They know that the right response will be greater interest and deeper involvement with you than in the past, not to mention greater support. Some relatives or friends may not want this responsibility, and some may not be able to handle it. They might make the effort, but they'll be in conflict.

☐ In addition to presenting a new responsibility when you tell someone you have this disease, you are taking on a new responsibility -- two, in fact:

The first is to make your best effort, in the face of disappointing reactions, not to take them personally. Even when people respond in unexpected ways, the ones who liked you still like you, and those who loved you still love you. Chances are that they will do their best for you, but, as noted, your news will stir up fears of their own. You want them to understand your situation, sure, but you have to understand theirs, too.

And that is your other responsibility -- helping those who react in unexpected ways to overcome or at least manage their own fears. There is only one way you can do so: by sharing the reality of what is happening to you and letting them know how you are responding to it. Some will listen with genuine interest, and others will simply not want to hear about it. You have to be sensitive to their needs, but you owe them at least an effort to put your situation into perspective.

In time, as you learn more, you may discover that your responsibility to your uninformed, misinformed or fearful friends has expanded. For many of those you meet, you will be the only man they have ever known who has faced prostate cancer -- or any other kind of cancer. You might ultimately feel impelled to become an educator on the subject, to sweep away some of the most frightening myths and explain the most important realities for those who are interested. (Be assured that you will become remarkably sensitive to just how much people want to know -- or prefer not to.)

How will you present your knowledge? In whatever perspective and tone of voice you find comfortable. My suggestion would be to start with reality. Do not duck the dangers and difficulties, but be sure to include the hopeful aspects of this condition. Remember that you are informing, not complaining. If a wry note comes easily to you, fine. It can reassure your listener that you're on top this situation, that it has not driven you to despair. When someone genuinely wants an explanation of the effects of hormone therapy on prostate cancer cells, for example, I tend to refer to these cells as "little bastards." The phrase accurately describes my feeling about them and seems to put listeners at ease.

You never chose to be especially knowledgeable about how prostate cancer works and about its effects on a man's life. The fact is, however, that you already know a lot. Even now, you probably have a better handle on the subject than most of your friends, and you will keep on learning. The subject may come up relatively infrequently. When it does, however, you will be in a wonderful position to be helpful. For better and worse, your credibility is high. Even if you do no more than remind a man to get his regular prostate checkups, you will be making a meaningful contribution.

SAYING IT

When you have just been diagnosed as having prostate cancer, knowing how to describe your condition to other people is the least of your concerns. You're worried or, just as likely, scared. You have homework to do and decisions to make. When you decide to tell someone about your situation, you'll have no trouble finding the words (but might find it hard to say them): "I have prostate cancer."

Finding the words will not always be this easy. You'll get the homework done, make the decisions, get treated and, with a bit of luck, come out the other end in good condition. At that point, describing your situation will become significantly more complex. The reason is the nature of the disease, itself. Any of the current, accepted protocols can produce a cure in some cases and significant control in others. Neither outcome, however, guarantees that all the prostate cancer cells have been removed or eradicated. Some of these cells are submicroscopic, capable of hiding from today's most sophisticated scans. What "cure" means is that the likelihood of their return or spread is small and, even if they should come back, years in the future. "Control" means a greater likelihood, still possibly years in the future.

As the effects of your treatment recede, you may discover that you feel about as good as ever -- maybe better because you've confronted this challenge and taken major steps to overcome it. Even if there should be a recurrence, don't conclude that all is lost. Looking at that possibility, Yoshiya (Josh) Yamada, MD, my radiation oncologist at Sloan-Kettering, once pointed out to me that "we have many arrows in our quiver."

Let's say that your treatment has been a success. Your PSA and other blood factors are what they should be, and the doctor's manual inspection has proven negative. You will continue to have your PSA and possibly other factors checked periodically, and the doctor will continue periodic manual inspections. Now, however, you will tend to approach these checkups with at least a touch of anxiety. You might even experience more than a touch, as I usually do.

Now assume that your latest checkup has been fine -- no sign of storm clouds in the sky. You're getting on with your life. The old "I have prostate cancer" no longer applies. It doesn't even come close. How do you define your condition to others at this point? Here are a few alternatives:

☐ **"I had prostate cancer."** We all want to say it, but are we sure the matter will be past-tense forever? More to the point, are we the least bit superstitious? Would we be more comfortable not making this statement flat out?

☐ **"I'm a prostate cancer survivor."** Well yes, you are. You have had the disease and dealt with it, and you're still here. *Survivor* is a good, powerful word, and lot of people use it. Cancer *survivorship* has come to be an accepted field of study because, happily, there are a lot of us. Still, I'm a little uncomfortable with the word. Like I *had* the disease, I'm a *survivor* smacks of having gotten it behind me for all time. When I apply the word to myself, I generally add *so far* or *up to now*. Superstitious? Maybe.

☐ **"I've had some experience with prostate cancer."** This statement makes sense if someone else has brought up the subject, and you have it in mind to contribute an insight. It might qualify you as an authority among your listeners. At the very least, it will indicate that you have a valid basis for expressing your views.

☐ **"I'm a prostate cancer victim."** I have never heard anyone say it and hope I never will. If someone is assaulted or robbed, that person is a crime victim. Someone can even be a victim of his or her own folly. It is worth noting that the word was first used centuries ago to signify the living creature sacrificed in a religious ceremony. By implication, the *victim* was blindsided, never had a chance, never had the opportunity to fight back. The event is over. You, on the other hand, do have a chance, and you are fighting back. I urge you to avoid this phrase.

☐ **"I've been treated for prostate cancer."** This approach strikes me as being demonstrably accurate and about right. The listener will most often interpret this statement as being in the past tense, though it can apply to the present, as well. It makes no claims about the future, positive or negative. "How did it go?" is sometimes the response, giving you the opportunity to talk about the subject briefly or at greater length, whichever you think is appropriate.

You will often be asked, "How are you doing?" or "How's it going?" Your answer will depend to some degree on who asks the question. If it is someone truly close, or a man who has faced prostate cancer himself, you will generally want to answer the question as accurately and sensitively as you can. Either one of these people will be genuinely interested in your response and might welcome details. If the questioner is a casual friend, fellow worker or acquaintance, on the other hand, the interest level is likely to be lower, and he or she might prefer not to get deeply into the subject. In this case, a simple "fine, thanks" or "feel great" is what the questioner most often hopes to hear. Unless you have an urge to reply in greater detail, an answer along these lines is a graceful, simple way to get past the subject. If the questioner should want to hear more, he or she will say so.

When I am asked one of these questions, I usually repeat the words of Dr. Yamada, who understands my case a great deal better than I do. At each of my regular visits to his office, currently at six-month intervals, I turn the question around and direct it to *him*: "How'm I doing?" The first time I did so, he said, "So far, so good." Those four words struck me as being an exact description of my status, marvelous news without any promises, and I still celebrate them.

How am I doing? So far so good. And thanks for asking.

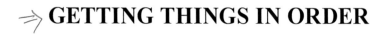# GETTING THINGS IN ORDER

The leader of my men's survivorship group, which includes veterans of all types of cancer, asked one of the participants the usual courteous question: "How are you doing?" This participant had been out of treatment for months and was well recovered, at least physically. His doctor thought returning to work would be good for him, and his wife agreed. The recovered man said he wasn't ready and even resisted the idea of working two or three days a week. "I need time to get things in order," he added. Another member of the group jumped on the statement. "Getting things in order," he said, "always sounds to me like what you do when you're getting ready to die."

No wonder. In countless television dramas, movies, plays, novels, short stories and jokes, a doctor, lawyer or clergyman says to some poor, doomed soul, "Well, guy, I hate to tell you this. It's time to get your affairs in order." That amiable suggestion, covering all those practical matters the condemned man has neglected up to now, has come to mean a lot more than it says: "You're finished, fella, probably pretty soon. There doesn't appear to be a way out. Unless you want to leave a mess behind, now is the time to get organized. You're not going to get another chance."

That interpretation of the phrase gets even more reinforcement. Many of the nation's leading banks, brokerage houses, accounting firms and insurance companies advertise professional help in getting our affairs -- at least our financial affairs -- in order. Fine, but they tend to label this service "estate planning." Most of us know that "estate" is the lawyer's word for what we're going to leave to our heirs; so once again "getting things in order" is directly associated with dying. And we're already dealing with a disease that not long ago was considered swiftly and unquestionably fatal.

So that outspoken group member had a point: This kind of organizing sounds much too negative, too final, a little like last rites. The fact is, however, that he was only half right. There are plenty of positive, life-oriented reasons for getting things in order and doing it sooner rather than later. When you have seriously disorganized aspects of your life, they are hard to ignore. You know you should deal with them, but "well, there are other priorities." Even when you're not thinking about these aspects, you have a nagging awareness of them. They come to feel like the shell that a turtle has to lug around except that the turtle makes good use of its shell every day. Life can never be perfectly neat, but it can certainly be richer and more enjoyable without these messy patches of disorder.

Like so many other practical issues, patches of disorder come in two forms, major and minor. The major ones bear on the most important aspects of your life (except, of course, for feelings and relationships): health, finances, shelter, lifestyle and sense of security. How "buttoned-up" are you in these vital areas? It is easy to determine:

1. Answer this question: "Do I *feel* buttoned up?" If the answer is no, you probably aren't.

2. List as many of your important documents as you can think of. Include the following if they apply: the deed or lease to your home or, in the case of a co-op apartment, your stock certificate and proprietary lease...insurance policies (life, home, car and/ or other property, liability, long-term care)...bank, brokerage or retirement-account statements...copies of income-tax returns for recent years, along with receipts and other backups for upcoming income taxes...children's birth certificates and health records... equipment leases...operating manuals for household appliances and other machinery...passport...Social Security and Medicare documents and healthcare proxy...credit card information... warrantees...will... marriage license and/or divorce papers... current bills...lists of key phone numbers and email addresses. There are sure to be other items, such as your safety box key, but you get the idea.

3. For each item on your list, answer these questions:
☐ Where is it located?
☐ How long would it take me to lay hands on it (or them)?

☐ How could someone else access it?

☐ Is it up to date?

4. Finally, answer these questions:

☐ Are there items on my list that I don't need?

☐ Are there items I do need that aren't on the list?

With the answers in hand, you will have at least a reasonable idea of how well or badly organized you are in some of the major parts of your life. If you see that your affairs are definitely not in order, you'll have at least a sense of what's required to get them straightened out.

The major patches of disorder count most, but the minor ones can be burdensome, too. Let me use myself as an example. My job is writing. As a result, I find myself surrounded by years' worth of file folders, some overstuffed, some with just a few pieces of paper. Because there is limited space in our apartment, the ones that don't fit in the file cabinet are piled up in drawers, in my clothes closet, on a windowsill and on a tabletop. These mostly visible file folders are not what my wife loves most about me.

The folders contain aging research notes, old newspaper and magazine clippings, first drafts, old letters, photographs and personal memorabilia. All my life, I have made sure I could ultimately find anything by the simple process of keeping almost everything. I've always had the confidence that comes from knowing that "it's here somewhere." The problem is that finding it is taking longer and longer. Worse yet, this mass of paper bothers me. Simply avoiding the time consuming, bothersome-but-necessary job of cleaning it up or transferring most of it to computer takes attention and energy.

The reason I got into this mess is that my whole generation has been living in a time of historic technological transition. I started work at a time when copies of office documents were produced by *carbon paper* (a tissue-thin sheet coated on one side with ink, which was transferred to the copy by the pressure of a metal typewriter letter at the same time that this letter was striking an inked ribbon in front of a sheet of paper known as *the original*. If the word *typewriter* is unfamiliar, please check the dictionary and celebrate your youth). All documents and folders were in the form of paper. The advent of the computer simplified my work but in no way cleared up the mess. Now, in addition to my accumulation of paper folders, I have boxes filled with unsorted disks.

I have never been good at discarding or deleting, but the time has come. Why? Because committing useless paper and electronic files to the trash bin will make it easier to find the useful ones. Because doing so will make more room for my next projects. Because reducing my paper and disk burden will simplify my life. Because the apartment will look better. Not least, because getting organized will mean I won't have to think about getting organized. I should have undertaken this task years ago.

My minor mess is paper. Yours may be different. Your closet may be stuffed with clothes you haven't worn for years, which the Salvation Army or a local thrift shop would welcome. You might have a garage filled with so many miscellaneous items that there is barely room for your car. Maybe you have a drawer filled with everything that belongs nowhere else, and you don't know for sure what's in there. You might have a shoebox or two filled with the photographs you've promised to put into albums. Minor patches of disorganization such as these are OK as long as they don't bother you. If they do, the time it will take to deal with them will be well spent. It will eliminate the bother.

Maybe you have always been well organized. If so, you've done well. For the rest of us, this is work we should have been doing routinely for decades -- whether or not prostate cancer turned up in our lives. Sure, getting our affairs in order, at least the major ones, might turn out to be helpful to our heirs at some point. At least equally important, though, is that doing so will be useful to us. Right away. In real time. Having our affairs in order will allow us to live more comfortably and to look straight ahead at new challenges, new opportunities and new pleasures.

The recovered man in the survivorship group? He went back to work a couple of months after the meeting. He also started devoting some of his spare time to getting things in order -- cheerfully, he told us later.

SEX

If you've turned to this section first, welcome! It's good to see that your interest in the subject hasn't flagged. You presumably want to know at least a few things right away. Fine, but be aware that the answers to your questions will ultimately emerge from your own experience. One of the important points made often in this book is that no two men are exactly alike, and neither are their prostate cancers. Generalities can be wonderfully useful, but they can't provide personal guarantees. That said, here are a couple of generalities that might serve you as a starting point.

☐ *Yes, there's likely to be a sex life in your future, possibly after a hiatus. Very few physical results of your treatment could rule it completely out. If all else fails -- and much can be done -- implants work. Psychological issues on the other hand -- high stress, high anxiety or depression, for example -- could get in the way. So could any sexual problems you might have had before you were treated. And, not least important, there can be a sex life in your future only if you want one.*

☐ *Your sex life will probably be different from the one you've been used to in small, medium or large ways. If you and your wife or partner are open to the changes, your sexual encounters can be intimate, exciting and richly satisfying.*

————————

While you're here, it might be well to take a look at the other side effect of prostate cancer treatment that most worries men: **incontinence**. *It's not unusual for patients to come out of their procedures with some kind of urinary difficulty. It can take many forms -- from a burning sensation...to a bit of leakage when they cough, laugh or lift heavy weights...to a more consistent inability to control the flow. In most instances, men regain their urinary control in a few weeks or several months after treatment -- especially if an advanced form of surgery, radiation or seed implantation has been employed.*

Meanwhile, there are medical ways to deal with incontinence and the usually temporary inconvenience it causes. Depending on the individual case, behavioral changes can help. So can pelvic exercises that strengthen the muscles that control the flow, as well as injections and surgery. All else failing, an implanted artificial sphincter can solve the problem once and for all.

Still, there's no ignoring the inconvenience, fear of embarrassment and self-image issues that even short-term incontinence engenders. We men have had no previous experience wearing absorbent pads and disposable underwear. "It's a damn bother," one man told me. "When I travel overseas on business, I have to pack a whole separate suitcase for my supply of disposable shorts." What struck me was that he was traveling overseas. He disliked the situation, but he was dealing with it. Ultimately, after many months had passed, his doctor inserted an artificial sphincter. He regained total control...and now travels lighter.

———————————

Back to the subject of sex. A closer look at it follows, but now might be a good time for you to start reading this book at the beginning.

When it comes to sex, nearly all of us have seen too many movies, and most of us have read too many books, from the classic novels to today's potboilers. Sure, they've told us a lot about the sexual attitudes and behavior of men and women, heterosexual or gay, but they've also left us with a lot of false impressions. For those of us who have faced treatment for prostate cancer, these misapprehensions can cause unnecessary concerns. Here are just a few of the movie-and-novel-generated ideas -- bolstered by television, magazines and gossip media -- that fall somewhere short of the truth:

☐ Great sex is for the young, beautiful and handsome.

☐ When partners are powerfully attracted to one another, erections are instant and orgasms can occur at very short intervals.

☐ Great sex just happens, and it happens fast. Thinking, not to mention planning, has no part in the equation.

☐ Great sex is serious business. Except for moans, groans, *yes*'s and ecstatic cries, it's also silent.

☐ Intercourse is the *sine qua non*, the *alpha and omega*, the be all and end all and the sole reason for being of sex. All women need deep penetration often and value it above all other things.

These common misconceptions can stir doubts in any man at or past middle age. Add the overlay of treatment for prostate cancer, and these doubts are amplified. First of all, a surgeon, radiation analyst or other medical practitioner will have been plying his or her trade at one of the two critical centers of the patient's sexual response system. (The other is due north, in his mind.) It's not unusual for men to worry about their potency under the circumstances, and anxiety, alone, can have a downside effect. Second, there will probably be discernible physical effects, temporary or longer term, on their sexual responses no matter which protocol they've chosen. These effects, as noted, can range from minor to major, with infinite variations in between. They vary widely among individuals, even when their prostate cancers have been treated in similar ways. They might require no treatment whatever, or treatment might be indicated. Once again, generalities don't serve as reliable predictors.

Here are some of the things that can occur as a result of prostate-cancer treatment. (If you are "watchfully waiting" as an alternative to treatment, none of them will immediately apply, but other troublesome issues might arise.)

Erections can be less rigid, may require more time and stimulation to take place and may require longer intervals "between engagements." Orgasms can come sooner or later than in the past, can be more or less intense than in the past, can produce relatively little semen or can be entirely dry. One *diagnostic* procedure (trans-urethral resection of the prostate) can result in retrograde orgasms, in which the fluid rushes "backwards" into the bladder (without harm and with only a minor change in sensation). There can be weeks or months of "downtime." Erections can become partial (reassuring but inadequate for intercourse) or completely impossible to achieve without medical intervention. The libido can fade away for a period of time. Or, for some men, the changes in response can be too small to perceive.

The list of possibilities can obviously be scary until you remember this: Many men don't lose their potency as a result of treatment, and most of the others can regain it. There are treatments that can help the great majority of affected men regain a rich, joyous sex life -- including erection and orgasm -- if they and, ideally, their wives or partners want it to be so. Should psychological factors intrude, mental health professionals who specialize in sexual issues can help. Should the need arise, your treating doctor can offer guidance for dealing with some of the most common forms of sexual dysfunction. If necessary, he or she can refer you to a specialist on staff, associated with the institution or known to it. Stick with reliable referrals and unmistakably valid medical or mental-health credentials. On the internet and in other media, many obscure sources offer erectile "treatments" and "cures" that sound too good to be true -- and might prove too good to be true. The stakes are too high to gamble.

Doctors generally approach post-treatment erectile dysfunction by first considering the simplest, least invasive approaches and thinking about the more complex and invasive ones only if the others won't suffice. In ascending order, the most common alternatives are drugs such as Viagra® (sildenafil citrate)...an external vacuum device or either of two forms of penile injection (both said by users to be far less distressing than they sound)... and, all else failing, penile implants. One or another of them can restore potency to most men when they are sexually stimulated. None is for everybody. Each treatment approach is based on the patient's erectile status, and each has its own characteristics and potential side effects. A qualified doctor's evaluation and decisions are absolutely necessary.

(For an excellent overview, I recommend *Sexuality and Cancer*, published by the American Cancer Society. In addition to offering invaluable information for men in relationships, it includes a useful section titled "The Single Man with Cancer.")

With the possible exception of religion and politics, no subject is ultimately more personal than sex. There are as many approaches to the subject as there are men. Recognizing that fact, let's take a closer look at the misconceptions presented earlier.

Great sex is for the young, beautiful and handsome. You know better, but when you watch American movies and television it's hard not to be influenced. The women who play romantic leads are, with a few delightful exceptions, young or just easing out of youth. Virtually all of them are stunning. The men are sometimes older but usually fall into the handsome or rugged category. (Foreign casting directors seem more comfortable with romantic leads who look like the rest of us.)

Sure, great sex is for gorgeous young people, but, as you almost surely know, it's not exclusively for them. It's for any two people who appeal to each other, want each other and, ideally, love each other -- regardless of their age and regardless of the extent to which they conform to the standards of casting directors and model agencies. Medical science makes it clear that there's no physical bar to a healthy man's enjoying sex throughout his life. Most of us in the prostate cancer fraternity are on the far side of youth, and we may not turn heads on the street, but we qualify.

When partners are powerfully attracted to one another, erections are instant and orgasms can occur at very short intervals. There was a time when it was so, peaking in our teens. A fleeting erotic thought was fully sufficient to stimulate an immediate erection. Now it's at least a little different. From the standpoint of sex, time seems to expand in two ways for many of us as we grow older: We need more time between sexual engagements if we're to reach orgasm, and we may need more time and stimulation to achieve an erection.

Treatment for prostate cancer can amplify these changes. It can even rule out erections for some of us, at least until we turn to medical or mental health professionals for solutions. (Remember, these solutions can be simple in many cases.) Still, even temporary impotence or partial impotence can be disturbing. Since puberty, most of us have relied on our ability to have erections as an important part of our identity. Any one of us might feel like "less of a man," though all the other aspects of our manhood are in place. This situation presents an obvious obstacle to couples, but it's by no means an insurmountable one. Even during this period, a couple can enjoy mutually exciting, fulfilling sex. (See the discussion of intercourse, later in this chapter.)

Great sex just happens, and it happens fast. Thinking, not to mention planning, has no part in the equation. We've all seen it in the movies or found it described in novels: Two lovers feel the overwhelming urge and tumble into bed, or wherever, as fast as they can. In films, the music usually rises along with everything else. Countless teenagers have fantasized this instant passage from wish to fulfillment -- this ability to "have sex whenever I want it" -- and some of us have experienced it. Many of us feel certain that the ability to respond immediately to an erotic urge, whenever and wherever, is an essential part of a truly exciting, satisfying sexual experience.

As it turns out, we're mistaken. An instant response may be absolutely delightful, but it's not essential. A man and his wife or partner can sometimes respond swiftly to a whim, but they can also think, plan and decide about when and where -- and still achieve a truly exciting, satisfying sexual experience. A bit of anticipation can be delightful, too.

If the very idea of planning seems unromantic to you, think about the most romantic moments you've ever had. Chances are that some advance thinking was involved in getting you to those moments. Planning can clear a space for spontaneity.

If it should turn out that you need even a small medical "assist" to achieve erections after treatment for prostate cancer, these observations take on special meaning. What's sex like when a pill, mechanism, injection or implant is part of the occasion?

"Just terrific, thanks," I heard one man say. "Different but fine." And a 67-year-old doctor, explaining that he'd ultimately had a penile implant after prostate surgery, told me that he "felt like a 22-year-old kid again." My mini-survey has been too small for statistical reliability, and reactions may not always be this good, but I've heard eminent specialists paint uniformly promising pictures in their lectures.

Great sex is serious business. Except for moans, groans, *yes*'s and ecstatic cries, it's also silent. No one can say enough about the moans, groans, *yes*'s and ecstatic cries that can occur. As you know, they signal the unimaginably intense experience of orgasm. It's beyond description, though the French come pretty close with the term *Le Petit Morte,* "The Little Death." Nothing is more serious at that moment. But from the first gentle touch, before the ascent to orgasm has begun in earnest, to some occasions after the climatic moment has taken place, there's more than enough room for playfulness, laughter, conversation and fun. (This fact may be old news to you. Does it always apply? Of course not. There are times in long established relationships, not to mention new ones, when passion and other emotions take precedence over any sense of fun. But it's a valid generality. In sexual matters there's very little that always applies.)

Why is it relevant here? Because, as noted, treatment changes most men's sexual responses at least temporarily -- maybe only slightly, maybe more substantially. If the changes are slight, so are the adjustments he has to make. He might need to make none at all. If the changes are greater, however, and if the man is part of a loving couple that cares about sex, there's mutual exploring to be done. There are experiments to pursue and new approaches try.

Most couples will approach these activities in their own way. Some may undertake them with studied seriousness. Others may find that they lend themselves to playfulness, humor and delight. Still others will combine these approaches or try others. Many will discern that verbal communication has become a more meaningful component of their sexual lives than in the past. Whatever the case, it will be helpful for them to remember that occasional disappointments can occur in any series of experiments. These disappointments are not failures. They're a normal part of a learning process that can, itself, be wonderfully pleasurable. They're to-be-expected steps toward the goal that all these couples share: to enjoy again the same sexual pleasure as before. Maybe even greater.

Intercourse is the *sine qua non*, the *alpha and omega*, the be all and end all and the sole reason for being of sex. All women need deep penetration often and value it above all other things.

NOTE: There's a chance that this section will have no relevance to you. It is for formerly potent men whose treatment has left them unable to achieve an erection even with a relatively simple "assist." And for most of them, the situation is temporary if they want it to be. Medical and mental health professionals stand ready to help them return to potency.

What would happen if I couldn't "rise to the occasion" and satisfy my wife? a man might wonder if treatment should leave him temporarily dysfunctional in this respect. *What would happen if this situation went on for months, even for a year or longer? Would she leave me? Would she take a lover?*

He probably won't ask these questions out loud, but you can't blame him for wondering. For one thing, the idea of the desirable woman who can't get enough coitus has been a male erotic fantasy for ages. She needs deep, vigorous penetration as surely as she needs air to breathe. She may exist, but there aren't many of her. She's anything but a representative of her gender.

For another thing, our worried man probably watches television and sees movies, witnessing numerous adulterous affairs on screen. He might know real-life examples personally or encounter them among the rich and famous in magazines or tabloid newspapers. If he reads literature, he can find women who stray from the marriage bed in classics from Aeschylus to Hawthorne, Tolstoy, Flaubert and Lawrence, all the way to Updike. No matter how secure this man's relationship may be, at least a whisper of uncertainty can sneak into his head. And it's partially justified. There are women who leave their husbands or long-time lovers under these circumstances, and there are women who take lovers (though it's doubtful that temporary impotence is the only reason in either case). They aren't representatives of their gender either.

Happily, most of us -- men and women, alike -- have more than one source of joy in our lives. Sex might be high on the list, but it doesn't stand alone. We also value our families, friends, homes, work, faith, communities, interests and much more. Also happily, our choice after prostate cancer treatment isn't either/ or. We and our wives or partners can have the other things on our list *and* a fulfilling sex life. In some instances, however, we might be obliged to set aside the long-held assumption that sexual encounters have to end in intercourse to be truly pleasurable. *If it doesn't end that way,* you might think, *it's all foreplay. That's fine as far as it goes, but it doesn't go far enough.* You're right. The foreplay you might be used to doesn't go far enough, but possibly it can go a lot further -- all the way to mutual orgasm. In other words, if you and your partner want to share sexual pleasure, you can.

Suppose you begin, patiently and without high expectations, with gentle, loving and ultimately sexual touching and stroking. Suppose your lovemaking should end there this time, without a climactic moment. You've shared a warm, intimate moment and given each other profound pleasure without intercourse. Now suppose that, on another occasion, you want to go further. Perhaps more of the same can bring you both to orgasm. If not, and if you both consider them desirable, you already know -- or can readily find out about -- those age-old techniques with the Latin names, as well as other techniques. (Yes, a man can have an orgasm without an erection.) If these approaches are new to you, be patient. They take practice to become as pleasurable and exciting as they can be.

And don't forget imagination and erotic fantasies. As you know, they can be among the most effective stimuli of all.

Two concluding thoughts on the subject of sex:

1. Try not to chastise yourself if you find that your libido isn't working well or seems to be hibernating. It's not an unusual phenomenon for men who've had the experience of dealing with prostate cancer. Depression can be at play. So can anxiety or simple worry. Any form of fear is a natural obstruction to sex, incompatible with the activity of your libido. Consider the much discussed "performance anxiety," for example. If you fearfully ask yourself, *Will I be up to it?* or *Will I be able to satisfy her?* the answer is likely to be *no.* The anxiety, itself, is the problem.

Obviously, just telling yourself not to worry won't help, but this thought might: You're not engaged in an Olympic sport here. Performance isn't the goal. Mutual pleasure is the goal, and that's within reach if you and your wife or partner both want it.

2. And here's one less thing to worry about: There appears to be no medical evidence that sexual activity increases the chance of recurrence of prostate cancer.

"BATTLING"

When media report that a celebrity has cancer, odds are that they'll say this celebrity is *battling* cancer. He or she is seldom *being treated for* cancer or *dealing with* it or *confronting* it. The word of choice is nearly always *battling.* Now there's nothing wrong with the word. It sets up cancer correctly as an enemy to be defeated and suggests that the only way to defeat it is by fighting it to the death – its, not yours. You can easily envision yourself wielding a broadsword, felling the hostile cells in massive numbers, never letting up until the last one has been obliterated. All well and good, but...

With luck, you'll come to a time when you are not doing much of anything in the combat. Let me explain.

There's no question that you're battling at the start and probably for many months thereafter. The process of choosing the right protocol will tend to occupy your thoughts every day and nearly every hour. Each telephone conversation or meeting with an oncological surgeon, radiation oncologist, urologist, general oncologist, internist or prostate-cancer survivor will feel literally like a life and death discussion. Then you'll plunge into your treatment program, showing up when and where you're told. You'll follow doctor's orders with a heightened sense of discipline. You might feel battle scarred by major or minor inconveniences, discomforts and/or fatigue. There might be some follow-up visits at short intervals after treatment. But then -- and it can seem suddenly -- there will nothing much left to do. You'll still face checkups a few times a year, but if the news is good the enemy will seem vanquished, possibly dead or possibly just unable to continue the fight right now.

You've been operating on a high-stress, high-energy basis for months, maybe even years. You've been a warrior, keyed-up and alert. Now, at last, you're home from your surgery or seed-implantation procedure or final external-beam radiation treatment, or your hormone therapy has concluded. You've done what had to be done, and your sense of moment-to-moment urgency wanes. There appear to be no immediate demands for action. This is a time for celebration, right? Unquestionably. You've earned it and have every reason to relish it.

Don't be surprised, however, if you also encounter another feeling at about this time -- a letdown or even sadness. It's by no means a universal reaction, but it happens to some men. Why? Perhaps it's because the combat on which they've focused for so long, the imperative that's driven them, has come to a seemingly sudden end. Perhaps it's because, with an easing of pressure, they can allow themselves to feel sad for the first time since they were diagnosed. Perhaps they're mourning the loss of their old, familiar assumption of immortality. Whatever the cause, feelings of this kind are not unusual, and -- for most men who experience them -- they pass. In time, these men become more involved in the lives they lived before treatment, rediscover their former interests and regain their zest.

For some men, however, there's more than sadness or mourning involved. Depression takes hold. It's a complex condition that can affect these men at any time -- long before diagnosis and before, during or after prostate cancer treatment. Only a qualified medical or mental health professional can diagnose it reliably. If a man should withdraw even partially from his close relationships, however...if the things that used to give him pleasure no longer do...if his motivation is diluted to the point that he's at least partially immobilized...if he has lost interest in the things he used to care about...if, in the words of one psychotherapist, his world has "turned from full color to low-contrast black and white," then he might well be clinically depressed. Unlike normal sadness, this condition tends not to pass without professional intervention. Happily, such intervention -- in the form of talk therapy or medication or both -- can work wonders. Suppose a man can't distinguish between sadness and depression? The old rule applies: When in doubt, check it out.

Can our doctors drive a stake through the heart of every one of our cancer cells? We certainly hope so, but neither we nor they can be absolutely sure they've done it. Prostate cancer recurs in some. On the basis of this uncertainty, many of us are motivated to battle on. But how?

Some men continue the fight by making prostate cancer research a central aspect of their lives. They spend hours on the internet, in public libraries and elsewhere to keep abreast of the latest treatment protocols, drugs, experimental programs and more. In some cases they become exceptionally sophisticated laymen on the subject. All presume that they are lining up the defensive strategies that might apply if the disease should ever attack them again.

Some battle on by pursuing complementary therapies, as noted in the chapter titled *Appointments*. They include changes in diet, exercise regimens, meditation, massage, reflexology, mind-body therapies, acupuncture and others. Given the approval of the cancer-treating doctors, these activities generally offer the immediate benefits of pleasure, relief of some discomforts and often an enhanced feeling of well being. Not least important, they give men a renewed sense of control over their lives. Though their treatments are over, these men are still *doing something* about their health.

Do these complementary therapies have a direct, beneficial effect on the disease? Medical opinions vary. There appears to be statistical and anecdotal evidence that some patients "do better" when they pursue complementary therapies, but no direct, causal links between them and prostate cancer cells have been scientifically demonstrated to date. NOTE: This statement should in no way be taken to mean that no such links exist. They might well exist. Some researchers at leading institutions suspect that changes in diet and other aspects of lifestyle might help reduce the chances of recurrence. They're determinedly pursuing proof of their hypotheses. Meanwhile, complementary therapies can unquestionably enhance the lives of many patients both physically and psychologically. Think about an exercise program that gives you extra energy...a nutrition plan that ultimately makes you feel better...a massage that reduces your tension...a meditation program that reduces your anxiety...or other activities. They may not strike you as battling, but consider this: Any one of them can contribute to a feeling of well being, and some of them (particularly the right diet, exercise and meditation) might, just might, help keep those tiny cells at bay at the same time.

How can you find reliable professionals in these specialties? Once again, your treating doctor is a good place to begin your search. His or her institution may offer one of more of these therapies in house. If not, the doctor can probably provide some guidance. So can support groups, friends and others. Be sure not to start any one of these activities without your doctor's approval.

Obviously, these two alternatives -- complementary therapies and ongoing research into medical treatments -- can be modified, mixed, matched or eliminated. Staying informed on the latest developments in cancer treatment, for example, can be achieved without spending untold hours on the task. The man who keeps up to date can also invest in complementary therapies, perhaps on a trial basis first. If one of these activities works for him, he can take advantage of it more often. The man devoted to exercise, meditation and/or or one of the other activities can follow cancer science less intensely if he wishes. The combinations are infinite.

There's a third alternative. It takes the focus off prostate cancer for long periods of time but doesn't ignore the disease. This option is simply getting on with your life as energetically and well as you can -- pursuing knowledge and enhanced general health simply as a natural part of the process. Living productively, lovingly and well may not be battling in the strictest sense, but it might be equally valuable.

Warriors don't fight at peak intensity all the time. They do so only when they have to.

A NEW NORMAL

"All I want to do is get back to normal."

The man who said it had completed a series of conformal, external beam radiation treatments and hormone injections just two weeks before. He was somewhat above 80 years old and a picture of health. A tall man, he moved easily. His skin was smooth and pink, and his bright blue eyes radiated alertness and intelligence. He taught at a law school in the Midwest and, for part of each year, performed pro bono legal aid services. He was used to spans of long workdays without a break. He was impatient to get back to work, but he was "tired all the time."

What this man meant by "normal" was obvious: exactly the way he felt during the weeks and months before he was diagnosed and treated. He was not yet aware that all prostate-cancer therapies tend to cause at least short-term fatigue. He had not yet learned that there might be some residual effects over the long term. Still, his evident will and fresh appearance suggested that he might come very close to his former state. There's a good chance that he will find himself happily working as hard and well as he did before. After all, men who have done so include:

- Former mayors of New York City and Los Angeles;
- A recent U.S. Secretary of State;
- The 2004 Democratic Party candidate for President of the United States;
- A manager of the New York Yankees;
- Jim Calhoun, coach of the national-champion University of Connecticut men's basketball team (who was back at the sideline just 16 days after his prostate surgery);
- Six personal friends of mine; and
- Hundreds of thousands of other men.

That said, the professor will almost certainly notice at least a few differences. He will discover that, subtly or more evidently, his *normal* has changed.

Being bright, this man will recognize that it has happened to him before. All the major events we encounter over the years tend to change our sense of *normal*. Here are just a few examples.

☐ Completion of our formal education;

☐ Marriage or other total commitment to someone else;

☐ Parenthood;

☐ A radical job or career change;

☐ Retirement;

☐ The loss of a loved one...

And, yes, by any measure the diagnosis and treatment of a prostate cancer combine as a major event. In varying degrees, this event is life changing. We may behave after treatment much as we did before, but we will never again be exactly as we were. There are two principal respects in which we are likely to notice departures from our previous *normal*:

Physical – Regardless of the treatment protocol you choose, you will probably experience one or more symptoms that are new to you, at least for a while. You will almost certainly not experience them all. They can include various kinds of soreness, changes in sexual capability, loss of urinary control, rectal bleeding and, perhaps most common, some measure of fatigue. These symptoms are distinctly individual. I have not yet met two men who had identical experiences. Keep in mind that many of these symptoms tend to be temporary, and there are effective medical responses to virtually all of them. Still, you might feel different after treatment -- maybe only slightly, maybe more substantially.

Psychological – You will have every reason to celebrate if your doctor says that your treatment has been successful or if he or she offers you at least a "so far so good." You may even find that, for the most part, you feel about the same as you did prior to diagnosis. Like that over-80 professor, you may be impatient to "get back to normal," and you may come very close. But you have experienced a loss of innocence. You've been handed an indelible reminder of your mortality. You've always known that no one lives forever, but this obvious reality never seemed so personally relevant before. This burnished awareness may rarely be, in advertising parlance, "top of mind," but it is almost sure to affect your perspective from time to time -- especially when any strange new symptom turns up. (If, on the other hand, mortality should be in your thoughts most of the time over a lengthy period, some counseling might be in order.)

Prostate cancer is clearly not the only thing that's affecting your sense of normality. All of us are growing older -- and at exactly the same rate. The very trajectory of our lives dictates changes. Some of these changes take place so gradually, over so many months or years, that we barely notice them. Then, one day, we do notice. *"Hey, I can ride my bike as far as I want to, across town if I feel like." "I can do this work." "I can carry much more responsibility than my boss thinks I can." "Why do I get so damn tired at four o'clock every afternoon?"* Epiphanies along this line don't come often, but for most of us they do arrive sooner or later. No one ever made the point better (as he did for so many points) than William Shakespeare. The following 27-line speech by Jaques in *As You Like It* has been given and quoted often for more than 400 years. Whether you're rereading it or coming to it for the first time, it is well worth your time.

"All the world's a stage,
And all the men and women merely players.
They have their exits and their entrances,
And one man in his time plays many parts,
His acts being seven ages. At first, the infant,
Mewling and puking in the nurse's arms.

Then the whining schoolboy, with his satchel
And shining morning face, creeping like snail
Unwillingly to school. And then the lover,
Sighing like furnace, with a woeful ballad
Made to his mistresses' eyebrow. Then a soldier,
Full of strange oaths and bearded like the pard,
Jealous in honor, sudden and quick in quarrel,
Seeking the bubble reputation
Even in the cannon's mouth. And then the justice,
In fair round belly with good capon lin'd,
With eyes severe and beard of formal cut,
Full of wise saws and modern instances;
And so he plays his part. The sixth age shifts
Into the lean and slipper'd pantaloon,
With spectacles on nose and pouch on side;
His youthful hose, well sav'd, a world too wide
For his shrunk shank, and his big manly voice,
Turning again toward childish treble, pipes
And whistles in his sound. Last scene of all,
That ends this strange eventful history,
Is second childishness and mere oblivion,
Sans teeth, sans eyes, sans taste, sans everything."

And there you have them, The Seven Ages of Man --
experienced (allowing a little space for metaphor) by the process of
simply staying alive, just hanging in there. Each of them obviously
reflects a radical change in what a man might, at any moment,
consider normal.

In other words, you're likely to encounter some changes without knowing whether they're caused by prostate cancer or simple chronology or both. As a case in point, I started noticing differences in my own performance long before my diagnosis. I was a runner, exceedingly slow but committed. (At the behest of my well-worn knees, I'm now a racewalker, even slower but still committed.) I always ended races far back in the middle of the pack or far forward in the back of the pack. I was proud of my ability to run a 9:20 mile once in a while, even though I could never put two such miles together, not to mention six-plus miles. I ran strictly to stay in shape and to enjoy being outdoors in all kinds of weather. My only competitor was myself, and I had been able to trim my times over the years.

Imagine my distress when the tide of minutes per mile started to run in the opposite direction. I trained. I pushed. But it really was a tide, and I was running against it. That was simply an effect of aging, well before prostate cancer became an issue in my life. After my treatment, the slowdown tide continued, but I've managed to stabilize my racewalking times. They're nothing to shout about, but they're OK. Running against the tide is part of the fun, but I know perfectly well that the odds over the long term favor the tide.

In the years since my radiation and hormone treatment, I've gotten past a few symptoms. The one that remains is a total energy drain that I experience most afternoons at about 4 PM, and it may have little or nothing to do with the disease or its treatment. I've fought this phenomenon and learned that a restorative nap makes more sense than pretending to ignore it, but this lesson is still hard to accept. Like many other boys, I was raised on words like *hard work, accomplishment, responsibility, achievement, improvement, going the extra mile* and *When the going gets tough*.... Inevitably, naps strike me as goofing off or quitting. They give me a vague sense of guilt. I'm slowly, very slowly, coming to accept the fact that a nap makes the rest of my day better. Grudgingly, I'm adjusting to this aspect of my new *normal*.

All of us cherish our ability to perform at our very best – or whatever has been our very best up to now. We know how well we can make love with those we love, play at our sports, work at our jobs and enjoy ourselves. These abilities and others are precious. There is every reason to fight to enhance them further, as we have in the past, or at least to maintain them. There is even good reason to carry on this fight longer and more effectively than anyone might have reason to expect. Alfred Lord Tennyson had the right idea when he committed his Ulysses – now getting on in years at home in Ithaca, his odyssey long behind him – "To strive, to seek, to find, and not to yield."

But…

If we live long enough, we slow down sooner or later -- whether from illness, accident or simply advancing years. Our strength and energy diminish. Some of our working parts begin to show signs of wear. Our physical reaction times slow. These phenomena may be subtle, but at some point we begin to notice them, even if those around us don't. There's nothing to be ashamed of here. How many NFL, NBA, NHL, MLB or USTA superstars in their 40's can you name? A few, sure. Not many. Even the almost imperceptible changes in their skills have pushed most over-40 athletes in new directions.

That's the physical reality, and there are exceptions even here. Think of Lance Armstrong, whose testicular (not prostate) cancer spread to his abdomen, lungs and brain. He not only regained his performance level but actually raised it enough to win seven consecutive Tour de France cycling championships, setting a new record. In the other aspects of our lives -- the ones that depend principally on our minds and feelings -- we have a good chance of doing as well as always...or even better.

Whatever the case, cancer changes us, however subtly. So do the passing years. What about just biting the bullet and accepting our new *normal*? Is acceptance a surrender? Maybe not – if you've tested your new limits to see if you can push them back to where they were or even beyond, tested them with everything you've got. At that point, acceptance might just be brave. It might free you up to find new ways to strive, seek and find and to yield little or nothing.

Should we battle uncompromisingly to defend all our present capabilities, exactly as they are right now? Should we press hard to increase them? Should we rage against any sign of diminution? Should we undertake a strategic retreat in one aspect of our lives while we advance in another? Should we just "go with the flow," letting whatever happens happen and making the best of it? Or should we keep all these options open, reacting to each situation as it arises? These questions apply not only to strivers but also to those who assign pleasure a higher priority than accomplishments. Might accepting the physical changes we experience actually heighten our pleasures?

There is no one-size-fits-all solution to this puzzle. In his mission to "get back to normal," our good, over-80 professor will eventually have to confront it. His response will derive from his character, from the man he has become over all these years. So will yours.

SYMPTOMS AND ASSUMPTIONS

Stuff happens. Curious symptoms can turn up...or not turn up. If they do, they may or may not include odd sensations you haven't experienced before -- twinges, aches, strange rectal or urinary-tract experiences or unfamiliar pains. You will almost certainly react to them as any sensible person in your situation would – with a sharp jolt of panic or gnawing fear or just simple, pervasive worry. It doesn't occur to you right away that these symptoms might have nothing whatever to do with cancer. You jump to the obvious conclusion and wonder what it will mean. Dr. Holland quotes from a poem by William Matthews in the *Atlantic Monthly*. "Once you've had cancer, you don't get headaches anymore, you get brain tumors, at least until the aspirin kicks in."

The problem -- and the good news -- is that your instant conclusion might be totally wrong. You did not, after all, spend four years in medical school and additional years in internship and residency finding out which conditions cause what symptoms. If you had, you would be a doctor, and even then you'd probably seek out another doctor to deal with your own case. You just don't have the data that can assault or obliterate your new fear. You have your imagination, but it is not usually on your side.

It has happened to me more than once. In one instance, a few drops of blood turned up in my urine on two separate occasions. *Whoops! What the hell is this?* I know that knowledge fights fear; so I pulled out my reliable *Merck's Guide* (layman's edition). Mistake (mine, not the book's). *Merck's Guide* touched on a few possible causes for this occurrence, one of which was cancer of the bladder. Terrific. Now I was really scared. I promptly called the nurse practitioner who works with my radiation oncologist. She assured me that the event could be the result of an infection or a delayed effect of my radiation. On the other hand, she said she couldn't assure me that the event did not signal an emergency. If this call didn't eliminate my fear, at least it eased my mind a little. Just knowing that something else, something relatively benign, could account for a scary symptom always helps.

Good doctors, nurses and other caregivers do not lie. They virtually always tell you the truth as they know it at the time. Without ruling out the possibility of serious trouble, they do what they can to relieve your mind -- sensitively and supportively. But the fact is that, when you call, they don't know enough about your new problem to offer an instant opinion. You know even less than that. Neither you nor your attentive practitioner will learn more until you are examined; so you make an appointment, ideally soon. In my case, a Tuesday phone call resulted in an appointment the following Friday. *There. That's good. I've been responsible. I've dealt with this situation in a timely way. Nothing more to be done until Friday. Now I can relax.*

No I can't. Not now anyway. It's Tuesday afternoon, and something seriously bad might be happening, and I won't have a clue about it until Friday. Even then, I may have to wait for lab results to find out. I realize that this might be nothing at all, but there's no way I can be sure. It's going to be a long three days.

Not necessarily. Unless you are subject to clinical depression or other serious psychological imbalances, it's worth noting that emotions about the most painfully difficult situations tend to come in waves. You can sustain your panic, your gut-gripping fear for just so long. Then, in ways the professionals may or may not fully understand, these terrors give way to other feelings. These feelings may not reach the level of pleasure, but they certainly offer welcome relief. I had responsibilities to meet that Tuesday, including several mindless ones outside the apartment -- letters and a package to walk to the post office, dry cleaning to retrieve and two cases of canned cat food to buy. Whatever else might be going on, these things needed doing.

I took the elevator to the street. It was a bright afternoon, warm for December. The first thing I noticed as I strode down the sidewalk was that my legs felt pretty good. Why not? I have been pretty assiduous about attending exercise classes at the Y three days a week and racewalking and running on other days. It seemed to be working. I could not have rediscovered that bounce walking from room to room at home. The place isn't big enough to reach full stride. But here, outside, stretching out, the feeling was good. The worry was still there, but I was not looking at it as hard as I had. In time, like a slow-moving cloud that slips behind a stand of trees, it was out of sight. Focusing on something you have to do, or just something you want to do well, is a wonderful distraction. My Friday appointment did lead to lab tests, and early the following week I was told on the phone that the results were negative. That positive news swept away the last clouds of that particular worry.

That was that, right? Problem solved. Maybe so, and if you believe it I say more power to you. For some of us, though, more is involved. Those odd symptoms that arise from time to time, our reaction to them, our age and the very fact of having a condition with *cancer* as its surname bring a hard fact into focus: We don't know what lies around the corner. That fact is nothing new, but we are more aware of it than we used to be. We have come face to face with a profound uncertainty. We have learned that it can sometimes unnerve us and push us off balance. The future looks a lot less reliable than it used to. We can go on living as we have in the past, and we do so for the most part, but we can no longer blissfully take the *long term* for granted. The difference may be subtle, but it is a difference.

When we are confronted with uncertainty, we are uncomfortable -- sometimes painfully so -- until there's a resolution. The uncertainty can range from the titillating to tragically painful: *Will my team win? Will I get the job? Does she or he love me? Will I be OK for the foreseeable future? Will she or he get through this operation OK? Will a war overwhelm us all?* Not every uncertainty can be resolved, certainly to our satisfaction. We have lived with that fact all along. Still, we crave resolutions. When they come, either we'll be a lot happier or we'll be saddened or worse. We'll have a more positive view of our immediate future, or we will know what we have to deal with. This time, however, there is unlikely to be a definitive resolution. A degree of uncertainty is an almost universal side effect of prostate cancer -- or any cancer for that matter. Do we have to live the rest of our lives on the edge of that razor blade? I don't think so.

First of all, we know that prostate cancer develops more slowly than other cancers. It is unlikely to smite us the way a stroke or heart attack might. We know that some physicians offer "watchful waiting" as an option. We know that treatments have continuously improved and that many men go on to live long, energetic and fulfilling post-treatment lives. Most important, we find out what our doctors have to say. If they have reason for optimism, so can we. If they are less sanguine, they will tell us what we need to know to move ahead. Depending on their conclusions, we can either relax or start organizing for action. At least we have a good idea of where we stand.

Fine, but we might face weeks or, more likely, months between appointments -- especially after treatment. That fact would be fine, too, except for our imaginations. They may very well kick in with doubts again, more often as the next appointment nears. Uncertainty is back. How can we deal with it? To start with, each of us will deal with it in his own way. If that way is the one that has worked for a lifetime, all the better. If it is not working for you now, here's a possible alternative:

If you have ever played poker, chess or bridge…or decided to change jobs…or served in the military…or invested in the stock market, you know that you sometimes have to make decisions without having all the information you'd like. What do you do? You gather as much information as you can in a reasonable period of time, and you think about it. Then you make an assumption and act on it. With a bit of luck, your assumption stands up, and the decision turns out to be the right one. Sometimes, as you learn more, you can make adjustments to the original assumption, and things work out even better. If that's the way you have coped successfully with uncertainty in the past, it will probably work out now, too.

There are two underlying assumptions available to men who have prostate cancer. They are implicit in that wonderfully ambivalent guideline many doctors provide as we undertake our search for a treatment protocol, institution and practitioner: "We're not dealing with a four-alarm fire here...but I wouldn't waste time." Put another way (in reverse order) the assumptions are these:

"I am going to live as if I don't have forever," or

"I am going to live as if I'm going to live."

The difference is not one of fact. It's one of attitude. We all know perfectly well that we're mortal. The question is not *if* but *when* mortality is going to catch up with us. So unless our doctors are prepared to give us projections of our individual spans -- and few, if any, are -- then we have no choice but to make our own assumptions. Should we now live our lives on the working assumption that our time might be running out fast, or should we adopt the view that we might just have long way to go? The hard data we're able to assemble is unlikely to point to a clear choice. We're left with personal preference as our only guide.

There's ample precedent for looking at life with a clear sense of its end. Back in the 17th Century, the English poet Andrew Marvell put it this way in *To His Coy Mistress:*

"But at my back I always hear
Time's wingéd chariot hurrying near;
And yonder all before us lie
Deserts of vast eternity."

The fact that Marvell was saying all this to hurry a young woman into bed takes nothing away from the sentiment. The great Satchel Paige, one of the most effective pitchers in the history of baseball, had staying young in mind but made the same point when he said:

"Don't look back. Something might be gaining on you."

Some men benefit from having their mortality in mind much of the time, aware that they "don't have forever." Knowing how evanescent life's experiences are -- how swiftly they pass and, in time, disappear entirely -- these men find little in life that's routine. Their experiences are heightened, just as a landscape is briefly made more vivid by the bright red, horizontal beams of light just before sunset. Birthdays, holidays and other special occasions can cause them a certain amount of emotional tumult. *Could this one be my last?* We know that some men prepare to fight any mortal threat by investing huge quantities of time into researching ways to overcome it. Others are depressed by any thought of The End -- sometimes to the point of virtual paralysis. Still others make important changes in their priorities (and may later be surprised to discover that they're living much longer than they expected).

On the other hand, men who focus on everything in their lives *except* its inevitable end, who live as if they're "going to live," go on with relatively few changes. Most of the time, they revert back to the old, familiar working assumption that they'll live forever -- or at least not worry about the alternative until the issue arises. They may have some panics, discomforts or deeply emotional moments from time to time, but the day-to-day texture of their lives doesn't change all that much. If they enjoyed life before their diagnosis, they most likely go on enjoying it much the same way after treatment

Which assumption, which *as if*, makes most sense?

Wait a minute, you might be thinking. *I've got a lot on my plate at the moment. Is this really a decision I have to make -- or even think about -- right now?*

No you don't. But sooner or later the subject of the rest of your life is going to come up, most likely after treatment, and this issue is going to come up with it. Even then, the *as if* you choose will probably be your own personal version of one or the other -- or possibly a combination of both.

As I see it, the choice reduces to this: Will we focus on the short term, with the undertone of sadness this focus implies? Or will we assume a longer term and respond to new and continuing opportunities for joy, pleasure, service and fulfillment? Despite my high Gleason Score, my personal choice is the second option as, in computer language, a default position. Why *default*? Because the assumption of a reasonably long future is the basis on which I choose to live, but I can't help recognizing that this assumption could be wrong. I may live with a view toward a reasonably long life, but I keep the possibility of a shorter one in my pocket. Sometimes I pull it out. Sometimes it comes out of its own accord.

I have heard scientists state that Man is the only animal that knows it is going to die. (They don't describe the interviews that led to this conclusion.) Whether or not this knowledge is exclusive to us, we humans are certainly aware of our mortality. Most of us don't spend a lot of time thinking about it, but our awareness has an inescapable implication: Being human demands consistent courage. It goes with the territory. If our species does, in fact, have an element of nobility -- and I believe it has, though a look at the world sometimes raises doubts -- it is because we live as we do, knowing what we know.

REMINDER

All of us are naturally focused on our cancer, but there's more than one thing going on here. We looked at this fact in the chapter titled *A New Normal*, but it has yet another implication: When too much is going on at the same time, we get the feeling that things are getting out of hand.

Though our disease can turn up relatively early in a man's life -- even in his 40's -- the vast majority of us are getting into advanced age. We're starting to notice that years of wear and tear have had an effect on our bodies. If we're active in sports, we might recognize that our muscle responses have slowed down. We are seeing faster than we can move. Frustrating. Or we might feel new stiffness in our knees, hips or other joints. Maybe we're experiencing difficulty hearing conversations or seeing traffic signs. If we have spent a lot of time in the sun, we might discover spots on our skin that we don't remember having seen before. Any number of orthopedic, gastroenterological, neurological, cardiological, ear-nose-throat, podiatric, dental or other symptoms could be arising.

We're not old, dammit, but odd things seem to be happening. Most of these developments go with the territory of the "golden years." We stay as active as we can, cling to our youthful spirit and eventually learn to live with these new conditions. We come to recognize most of the signs of aging and generally accept them. (My mother, then in her 80s, used to say, "You have to be a good sport if you get old.") But we have experienced a kind of cancer. Now, when we feel something really strange in our bodies, something we don't remember having felt before, many of us wonder if this is a sign of what we fear most. Our heartbeat quickens and palms moisten. We need to know as soon as possible if something *else* might be responsible. At this level of anxiety, there is every reason to pursue the answer. As suggested before, when in doubt, check it out.

Obviously, our experience with prostate cancer does not exempt us from other medical concerns. We can generally deal with one disease effectively, even with grace. When another medical problem comes up at the same time, however, it is troublesome. No general wants to be surprised by finding his army in a two-front war. And if a second new problem is troublesome, the addition of a third can be even worse. It can spark a tremor of fear and a sense that "it's all breaking down."

I'd guess that most of us have, over the years, found ourselves dealing with a major problem at any given moment of our lives. We're used to doing so. It's normal. Everything's under control. When two or three major problems occur simultaneously, however, our sense of normality goes out the window. In a war or any other situation that confronts us with several dangerous, complex, high-stakes battles -- all at the same time -- our problems seem to increase exponentially. There are moments when our situations seem totally out of control. We feel overwhelmed.

Prostate cancer has become part of our lives. Even if no other serious challenge arises, it is easy to wonder just how much control we have over our own futures. *How do we live with this thing?* The next chapter takes a look at some answers.

GETTING YOUR ARMS AROUND IT

Most of us have had a sense of control for as long as we can remember. We've all been presented with problems, sometimes big ones, and we've dealt with them. We've gotten a handle on them, decided what to do and then done it. Sometimes we've asked for and received help. Whether totally successful or not, we've taken charge of these situations. That's what we do, and that's what we're doing now as we face prostate cancer.

With most physical problems -- including accidents, sicknesses and diseases -- we move steadfastly from problem to solution. We may not always travel swiftly, but we usually get the job done.

We get a broken bone set, and it's as good as new, maybe better, seldom worse. We get shingles, take the prescribed medications and pain relievers and finally, after a while, we feel fine again. We feel even better when the doctor explains that this disease rarely strikes twice. Even when we have our chest opened for open-heart surgery or a coronary bypass, most of us recover, get into rehab, change our diet and exercise regimen and do everything else we can to make sure this damn thing never happens again. Then we put the matter behind us and get back to our normal lives -- or as close to normal as we can. Case closed. Glad that's done with.

This time it's different. With prostate cancer, we move steadfastly from problem to solution, at least for now. You read that right -- *solution, at least for now.* These mean, little invaders we're fighting, these little bastards, are never going to be destroyed with certainty forever. We may kill some and knock out others for years or even decades to come. They might never return in our lifetime, but, as one urologist says, "They want to come back." Prostate cancer is a chronic disease, and it can metastasize.

All of us are aware that we have never had total control over our lives. We're subject to the effects of wars, economic downturns, natural disasters, accidents, communicable diseases and other outside sources of danger. Still, most of us build a zone of psychological safety around ourselves and our families. It's not perfect, but within it we feel we are pretty much in control of what happens. This time, however, the danger is inside us. It may be a small danger after treatment, but there is no guarantee that has gone away forever. Unless we die of some other cause first -- which, depending on our ages, is not unlikely -- it could strike again.

This breach of our safety zone can rattle our sense of control. Most of us respond promptly to the imperatives -- to select and secure the treatment we determine to be best for ourselves... to report for our post-treatment checkups and work with our oncologists or other doctors to deal with whatever comes up... and to pursue any complementary therapies or lifestyle changes we think might help (so long as our doctors don't disagree). Depending on the protocol we choose, the initial treatment can take weeks, months or years. But the process doesn't end with the initial treatment. Periodic checkups lie ahead, perhaps semi-annually, maybe more often, sometimes less. Unless you suffer what the doctors call a relapse or recurrence -- in which the little cells reappear, possibly somewhere else in your body -- these checkups will continue for the rest of your life.

In other words, we all have a problem that might never be totally resolved. The word *cure* does not apply in the way we usually mean it. Cure, as used in many cancer-treating institutions, means being cancer-free for give-or-take five years after the treatment. That's no small achievement for a disease that had few long-term survivors just a couple of decades ago. If you reach that point, the odds are good that your prostate cancer will never trouble you again...but it could.

How can we adjust to life under this Sword of Damocles? Damocles, himself, offers no answers. He was a member of the ruler's court in Sicily in the fourth century B.C.E. and spoke expansively about how fortunate the ruler was. The ruler decided to teach Damocles the lesson that the life of power was precarious, invited him to a banquet and seated him under a sword suspended by a thread over his head. We know how Damocles got into this situation, but history doesn't tell us how he managed to get through dinner.

How can we get our arms around this new, possibly small but permanent uncertainty and still get on with our lives? If you haven't addressed this question before, you'll soon discover that you're in challenging territory. You'll almost certainly gain a new appreciation for the good things in your life. At the same time, you're bound to give thought to the bad things that can happen, including dying. These are the things they talk about in churches, synagogues and mosques, the issues Buddhists and Hindus contemplate, the giant concerns that probably led to all belief systems. This is the country philosophers inhabit, the land where people seek meaning. How can we simple laymen regain our sense of control? How can we gain perspective, even *think* about this situation?

As we discover so often when prostate cancer is involved, there is no single answer. There are many answers. Each man finds the one that works for him -- often with the help of spouses, friends, therapists, men or women of the cloth, other men who have been treated for prostate cancer, authors or others. Ultimately, our life experience leads each of us to his own solution. Once again, it's every man for himself.

Following are some of the answers I have heard. Most relate to prostate cancer. Some involve other cancers.

"It's like a boulder in the road."

"It gets in the way. I was doing fine -- happy at home, great wife and kids, good job -- and then this happened. It's like a boulder in the road. You've got to get around it, and you can't think about anything else, even if it takes years. And when you finally do get around it, you're still not past it. You have to drag it along with you wherever you go -- like a ball and chain. I'm getting used to it, but it's still heavy."

"The way I see it, God is testing me."

"My doctor thinks my cancer might be spreading. He sent me for some scans earlier this week, and I'm waiting to hear from him. The way I see it, God is testing me. I've been doing everything I'm supposed to about this cancer, everything. I'll keep doing that. I think that's what God expects of me. I think he expects me to do it without a lot of complaining and feeling sorry for myself. That's part of the test. I don't know how it's all going to come out, and the docs don't say. It's in God's hands."

"I sometimes describe cancer as an uninvited stranger in your house." (*From a mental health professional*)

"In my counseling groups, I sometimes describe cancer as an uninvited stranger in your house. He can be terribly dangerous to you, and he'll never leave. He can hide in a dark corner and become almost invisible for many years -- maybe until you move -- but he could come back at any time. How do you learn to live with this stranger? Do you try to get to know him better so you can build the strongest possible defenses? Are you aware of him all the time? Do you pretend he's not there except when you're forced to notice? Can you live pretty normally from now on? Or do you have to develop new ways to think? It's hard enough to wrestle with these questions when they involve a stranger in your house, but the answers can also apply to the reality of cancer in your body."

"I started to wonder if it might not better to think about the ways body, mind and spirit are *separate*."

"Yoga and yoga meditation -- I've practiced them for years -- they teach us that we're unified: body, mind and spirit. One being. Each aspect affects the other two, and you can't separate them. I've totally believed that for a long time, even now, but... When I got prostate cancer, I started to wonder if it wouldn't be better to think about the ways body, mind and spirit are separate. This thing sure affects my mind and spirit, but those are both basically OK. It's the body that's the problem. It's as if I'm driving a car, and my mind and spirit are just fine, thanks. But there's something seriously wrong with the car. I take it to the best mechanic in town. He does the work and says he's fixed the problem as well as it can be fixed. Might never happen again, but you can't be completely sure. Meanwhile, the car should run just fine; so I can keep on driving. I'm doing that now. Problem is, if this mechanical problem should ever come back, it might be harder to fix, and I can't get a new car. I try not to think about that."

"When it gets to me, I reach into my bag of tricks."

"When it gets to me, I reach into my bag of tricks. I don't think one thing is enough. Sometimes I just get away from what I'm doing and take a long walk. Sometimes I drive out to the airport and get a shoeshine. Sometimes I take in a movie, even a bad one. Almost any movie can get you out of yourself. I might sit in the back of a church -- doesn't matter what kind -- and pray.

It's always quiet there. Or I'll get together with a couple of friends for lunch or a drink after work, and we'll talk. Not about cancer. About anything that comes up. I always feel better afterwards."

"I don't think about it."

"I don't think about it. Honestly. I got it treated. My doctor said it all went well. I feel great. End of story."

"Maybe trouble sort of defines people. Maybe how I'm dealing with this thing right now is defining me."

"I suppose we all wonder who we are sometimes. At least I do. I can tell you about my family and my job without even thinking. Music I like, movies I like, teams I root for, my house, car, where I went to school -- all that stuff is easy. But talking about the deeper stuff -- you know, that's a lot harder. I've noticed that when people are under pressure, like when they're trying to handle a tough break, that's when you get to know what they're really about. We're all pretty much the same until that happens. Then you start to see the differences. Maybe trouble sort of defines people. Maybe the way I'm dealing with this thing right now is defining me."

"I allow myself to worry as much as I like and even to stumble into abject terror -- but only during the last month before my checkup."

"My checkups these days come every six months -- you know, PSA and testosterone readings, the manual exam, a conversation about the how I'm feeling. Now there's no way I'm not going to worry as the date approaches. It's bound to happen anyway; so I give myself permission. I allow myself to worry as much as I like and even to stumble into abject terror -- but only during the last month before the checkup. The way it's worked out, I've avoided the worrying until the last couple of weeks and had moments of terror only in the last day or two. That gives me at least five months to focus on the things I care about. Call it distraction or denial, if you like, but this approach works for me. It lets me live without the drag of thinking about prostate cancer all the time."

"As soon as you wake up, celebrate."

"As soon as you wake up, celebrate. A lot of people didn't make it through the night. It has been a good day already."

And one more, one that I heard myself say:

"*ne cede malis*"

"Everything helps -- people you love, good doctors, religion, philosophy, friends who actually understand. For me, there are also three words. They're the motto of the school I went to all those years ago, and I've carried them around ever since. They're in Latin: *ne cede malis*. Literally they say, 'Don't give in to difficulty' or 'don't quit.' They mean even more. They're part of a message the gods sent to Aeneas in *The Aeneid* of Virgil. The translator -- his name was John Edmund Barss -- said that 'they were really meant to hearten a man facing a fight whose end he could not see.' Here's the full translation of those three words.

" 'In difficulties flinch not thou,
But meet them with a stouter heart

111

Than destiny herself shall give thee leave.' "

These approaches are only a small sampling. They are *right* only to the extent that they work for the individuals who are taking them. They represent just a few answers to a question we all share: How can I live -- positively and happily -- with the reality of my prostate cancer?

And now, if you haven't yet developed your own answer, it's your turn.

NOT THE END

You and I are on two separate journeys. They're unique, individual to each of us. Still, we have things in common, especially one very important thing. I've shared what I've experienced and learned about this thing, and you've been gracious enough to come this far with me. Now it's time to close. Most books wrap up with a simple THE END, but that "one very important thing" rules out the usual closing. With my warmest good wishes to you on your own journey, I prefer to leave it at this:

TO BE CONTINUED

ABOUT THE AUTHOR

DAVID S. WACHSMAN is an independent public relations and communications consultant. He has worked often with the National Executive Service Corps. He was for 41 years owner and president of the New York public relations agency that bore his name. Its national and international clients included IBM, the Oxford University Press, Absolut Vodka, Chase Manhattan Corporation, Dean Witter Discover, Sealtest, Evian Water, John Wiley & Sons, The Office of Marcel Breuer, The American Society of Landscape Architects and numerous television productions including The American Short Story (PBS, two seasons), Mystery! (PBS, first two seasons), Too Far to Go (NBC), and Middletown (PBS). He graduated from Loomis School, holds a B.A. degree from Yale University and is a U.S. Army veteran. He is married and father of two sons. He was diagnosed with prostate cancer in the fall of 2000.

CPSIA information can be obtained at www.ICGtesting.com
Printed in the USA
BVOW020054041211

277374BV00004B/1/P